Coping With Peripheral Neuropathy

Coping With Peripheral Neuropathy

✦

How to handle stress, disability, anxiety, fatigue, depression, pain, and relationships

Scott I. Berman MD, CIDP (sufferer from chronic inflammatory demyelinating polyneuropathy)

iUniverse, Inc.
New York Lincoln Shanghai

Coping With Peripheral Neuropathy
How to handle stress, disability, anxiety, fatigue, depression, pain, and relationships

iUniverse books may be ordered through booksellers or by contacting:

iUniverse
2021 Pine Lake Road, Suite 100
Lincoln, NE 68512
www.iuniverse.com
1-800-Authors (1-800-288-4677)

Because of the dynamic nature of the Internet, any Web addresses or links contained in this book may have changed since publication and may no longer be valid.

ISBN: 978-0-595-44967-5 (pbk)
ISBN: 978-0-595-89286-0 (ebk)

Printed in the United States of America

The information, ideas, and suggestions in this book are not intended as a substitute for professional medical advice. Before following any suggestions contained in this book, you should consult your personal physician. Neither the author nor the publisher shall be liable or responsible for any loss or damage allegedly arising as a consequence of your use or application of any information or suggestions in this book.

Dedicated to my wife, Jennifer,
And my children, Rachel, Joshua, and Jordan
For all their love and support,
And for helping me to learn how to cope.

Special thanks to: Debbie Dawson RN, Eileen Evans
(Lehigh Valley Peripheral Neuropathy Support Group
Leader), Terry Heiman-Patterson MD, Artis "Pete"
Palmo Ed. D., Susan Matta DO,
Robert Coni DO, Zachary Simmons MD, Paul Berman
(for editing)

**Proceeds from the sale of this book are donated to:
Good Shepherd Rehabilitation Hospital**

Good Shepherd Rehabilitation Network, based in Allentown, Pennsylvania, is a nationally recognized rehabilitation leader, offering a continuum of care for people with physical and cognitive disabilities.

Good Shepherd specializes in the use of assistive and rehabilitation technology to maximize the function and improve the well being of its patients and clients. Leading-edge technologies are used throughout the Good Shepherd network. Children with disabilities are fitted with communication devices in the Pediatrics Program; long-term care residents benefit from environmental control units throughout their complex; clients of the Harry C. Trexler Center for Assistive Technology are custom fitted for high-tech wheelchairs and adaptive driving equipment, and work with state-of-the-art alternative and augmentative communication devices and electronic aides to daily living.

Good Shepherd offers specialized programs in stroke, orthopedics, brain injury, spinal cord injury, pediatrics, amputation and more. The organization operates inpatient rehabilitation hospitals, outpatient sites, a long-term acute care hospital, long-term care homes for people with severe disabilities, an independent living facility, a Work Services division that provides employment training and job placement for people with disabilities and a lifestyle products store called Rehability. Good Shepherd is also the majority owner of a joint venture with the University of Pennsylvania Health System (UPHS) in Philadelphia, Pennsylvania. Beginning in 2008, Good Shepherd Penn Partners will serve as the post-acute care provider for UPHS.

Good Shepherd, which is affiliated with the Evangelical Lutheran Church in America, was founded in 1908 when The Rev. John and Estella Raker invited a disabled orphan named Viola into their Allentown, Pennsylvania, home.

For more information, visit www.goodshepherdrehab.org. The phone number for general information is 1-888-44-REHAB (73422).

Contents

Foreword: Coping with Peripheral Neuropathy

This book is designed for the patient who has already been diagnosed with one of the many forms of peripheral neuropathy. It is designed to be an overview of the issues you will face and ways to cope with them. As you will see, peripheral neuropathy affects people in many more ways than simply affecting their peripheral nerves.

Peripheral neuropathy patients need to be aware of how to get a clear diagnosis when many neuropathies appear similar. They need to find some way to deal with the diagnosis. They need to learn to adapt to weakness, cope with chronic pain, and stand up to fatigue. They need to deal with the anxiety and depression that comes along with a chronic disease. They need to deal with changing roles, such as job loss, and changing relationships with spouses and children. Finally, they need to know how to get the different kinds of help they will need. This booklet covers each of these areas briefly, with a focus on "hands-on" advice for coping, and explanations of how one illness can interfere with so many parts of your life.

Peripheral neuropathy, or any chronic incurable disease, has profound changes in how you view life. Have you ever had a dream where you're falling endlessly, spinning out of control, desperately trying to grab on to anything or anyone for safety? You wake up, heart pounding; sweating, relieved that everything is all right. When I have this dream I awaken, briefly calm down, and then break into a sweat all over again as I realize that even awake, everything is *not* all right. However, with time, patience, support from family or friends, a willingness to get educated about your illness, and a willingness to accept treatment, most of us can learn to cope, and even to enjoy some parts of our lives.

This book is a work in progress. I want fellow peripheral neuropathy sufferers to send their stories, tips for coping, ideas, and resources, and I will incorporate them into future editions, giving credit to each contributor. I hope that this will eventually lead to a book that is a comprehensive "user's guide" to coping skills. A number of other books about peripheral neuropathy are already available, such as Senneff's *Aching Soles and Painful Toes* and *Aching Soles and Other Woes*, which cover treatment options in depth. While this book has some overlap with others, I hope to cover some new ground in the coping skills department.

"You can't always get what you want … but if you try sometime, you just might find, you get what you need"—the Rolling Stones. When I was a first year psychiatry resident one night on call the police brought in an old homeless man. He was dressed in torn clothing, filthy, sickly, and upset about being taken off the street. I interviewed him and he told me that the government was out to get him. He told me he wanted to shoot President Reagan. Most of the experienced staff felt that he had no real chance of harming the President; they doubted he could even recognize the President. But being a conscientious resident, I called the number for the Secret

Service. They told me to hold on to him, and they would send an agent out to interview him. I felt bad for the old man; I doubted he would harm anyone but I feared that he would become violent when I told him that a government agent had to see him. I walked into his cubicle and he demanded, "I want to talk to the FBI!" Thinking fast I said, "I can't do that but I can get you the Secret Service." He was happy with this and after having coffee with the agent he calmed down and let me admit him to the hospital.

When I graduated from Brown, President Swearer told us that an educated person was "one who could meet appointments that were never made." Very often this came to mind during my years of handling crises as a psychiatrist. Little did I know that the toughest appointment I never expected would be my own illness.

I
Getting a Clear Diagnosis

It began as a small spot of numbness on my left foot near the big toe, and my doctor didn't think it meant much of anything. After I tore a ligament in my left knee in an accident, the numbness and tingling started going up my leg. My orthopedic surgeon told me rather defensively "that it wasn't anything he did" and sent me for my first EMG, which came back normal. Some months later my family doctor ran some blood tests, and finding no cause for the numbness, sent me to a neurologist.

Over the next months I had another EMG, a spinal tap, evoked potentials, MRI of the brain and entire spinal cord, CAT scan of the chest, abdomen, and pelvis, and a bone marrow biopsy. I had so many blood tests ordered that one day the lab tech had to draw 30 tubes at once; she insisted I have juice and cookies before I stood up so I wouldn't faint. My abnormal EMG in my legs and the high protein in my spinal tap pointed to an inflammatory neuropathy, perhaps CIDP (Chronic Inflammatory Demyelinating Polyneuropathy). I was sent off to Johns Hopkins to see a subspecialist. I was told my diagnosis was absolutely wrong, and that it wasn't CIDP, although the specialist didn't know what it was. Even a nerve biopsy didn't shed much light. I was tired, and worried. I went to see my hometown neurologist. "Bob," I asked, "am I going to be chronically ill or is this thing going to kill me in short order? Am I 'circling the drain?'" Bob thought this was a good question so he sent me for a PET scan to look for hidden cancer, which thankfully was not found. Two years and two more specialists later, even the Hopkins neurologist thought I really did have CIDP, just an unusual variant that didn't respond much to treatment. So far I have had 6 EMGs, 6 spinal taps, 5 sets of brain and spinal cord MRIs, multiple other repeat tests, and I have about 11 doctors treating me for CIDP, its complications, and other illnesses I got along the way.

Peripheral neuropathy refers to a large group of diseases, all of which affect the peripheral nerves (nerves after they come off the spinal cord). Peripheral neuropathy is not in and of itself a diagnosis. There are a great many causes of peripheral neuropathy, and getting an accurate diagnosis in essential. The fundamentals of diagnosis are well described elsewhere (for example, Latov and Donovan: *Understanding Peripheral Neuropathy* available through The Neuropathy Association at www.neuropathy.org). This chapter focuses on what you need to know as a consumer.

The central nervous system comprises the brain and the spinal cord. Peripheral nerves coming off the CNS consist of sensory nerves, motor nerves, and autonomic nerves. Sensory nerves carry position sense and vibration, pain and temperature. There are large fibers (which carry position sense) and small fibers (pain and temperature), which can be myelinated (coated with a special sheath) or unmyelinated. Motor nerves control muscle movement. Autonomic nerves control involuntary processes such as breathing, heartbeat, and blood pressure. By convention, peripheral neuropathies consist of sensory or mixed motor sensory neuropathies, while nerve-muscle disease is termed "neuromuscular." There is a fair bit of overlap.

There are multiple ways to organize the hundreds of causes of peripheral neuropathy. The onset may be fast or slow. It may be just one side or symmetrical. The EMG can help distinguish between axonal damage (damage in the nerve cell) and demyelination (loss of the sheath covering the nerve cell. There may be proximal (closer to the body) or distal (hands or feet) involvement. Figuring out the cause of neuropathy can be very confusing, which is why neurologists devise ways to organize their thinking and narrow down the field. (see *An Algorithm for the Evaluation of Peripheral Neuropathy*, Ann Noelle Poncelet, MD, American Family Physician, Vol. 57/No. 4 (February 15, 1998) Common neuropathies in developed countries include diabetic neuropathy and alcohol induced neuropathy. Worldwide, the leading cause of neuropathy is leprosy.

Some causes of neuropathy:

Hereditary: Charcot-Marie-Tooth disease

Toxic: lead, arsenic, mercury, gold, thallium, carbon monoxide, glue sniffing

Infectious: HIV, Lyme disease, leprosy

Inflammatory: Guillan-Barre, CIDP (chronic inflammatory demyelinating polyneuropathy), MMN (multifocal motor neuropathy)

Paraneoplastic: secondary to lung cancer, lymphoma, myeloma, others

Drug induced: long list of drugs

Endocrine: diabetes, hypothyroidism

Nutritional: alcoholism, B-12 deficiency, folic acid deficiency, thiamine deficiency

Connective tissue disease: Rheumatoid arthritis, Polyarteritis nodosa, Systemic lupus erythematosus, Churg-Strauss vasculitis, Cryoglobulinemia, Sjogren's syndrome

Compressive/traumatic: carpal tunnel syndrome

First, you are going to need a neurologist. While your family doctor may be treating the underlying cause, such as diabetes, it is not reasonable to expect your primary physician to be an expert in peripheral neuropathy. If the diagnosis is not obvious after seeing a neurologist, then you should seek a consultation with a sub-specialist in peripheral neuropathy or neuromuscular diseases (there is a lot of overlap).

Expect and request adequate diagnostic testing. This testing should include blood tests for a wide range of disorders including B-12 deficiency, HIV, Lyme disease, thyroid disease, kidney disease, autoimmune disorders such as Sjogren's syndrome, and tests for antibodies that tell you that your body is attacking itself. There are also tests that are markers for a possible cancer as the cause of the neuropathy called "paraneoplastic antibodies." "There are tests for abnormal proteins in the blood and urine, called paraproteins, which can be related to neuropathy. For more details on testing visit the neuromuscular web site at the University of St. Louis at www.neuro.wustl. edu/neuromuscular, and the Athena diagnostics website at www.Athena.com. There are genetically transmitted hereditary neuropathies such as Charcot-Marie-Tooth disease, and genetic testing, while expensive, may be important. This is especially so if there is a question of more than one affected member of a family or a concern about transmitting the disease to a child.

Virtually everyone should have an EMG/NCV (electromyography and nerve conduction velocity) test. This is a lovely procedure where electric shocks are administered to your arms and legs and a computer measures whether your nerves conduct the signal at the proper rates. Then little needles are placed in various muscles to see if your nerves stimulate the muscles correctly. This testing is somewhat uncomfortable, but most people can tolerate it, and it is essential to getting a proper diagnosis, as well as following changes over time. MRIs of the brain and spinal cord should be expected to rule out central nervous system disease, and are generally tolerable. You can ask for a mild sedative if you are claustrophobic.

A spinal tap can tell a lot about inflammation and is not terribly uncomfortable if done by a well-trained neurologist. You may get a headache, but lying down for several hours after and lots of fluids usually help. The presence of increased protein can indicate inflammatory disease, and the presence of white cells (and bacteria) can help look for infection. Multiple other tests including tests for Lyme disease and neurosyphilis can be run on spinal fluid.

You may also be sent for "evoked potentials." These are tests where recording electrodes are placed on your head to see how your brain reacts to different stimuli. *Visual* evoked potentials are done by staring at a screen with various patterns, while *auditory* evoked potentials stimulate the brain with sound, and *somatosensory* evoked potentials are done by giving electric shocks to the arm and leg (similar to an EMG, except this time the brain's response is recorded).

Your goal as a patient should be to make sure that there is a fair bit of diagnostic certainty about your diagnosis. Tell your doctor you will do whatever tests are necessary or go to any sub-specialists needed to be clear about your problem. Remember, neuropathies can get worse with time, so getting a diagnosis early on is important.

Unfortunately, a significant percentage of neuropathies are idiopathic. This is a fancy word for "of unknown cause." The chairman of neurology at my medical school used to say that idiopathic meant "that we were such pathetic idiots that we didn't know what was wrong."

If the cause of your neuropathy is not immediately clear, you must at least know that potentially dangerous or fatal illnesses have been ruled out. These include "paraneoplastic neuropathies," which are neuropathies caused by cancer cells that put out harmful chemicals. Neuropathy has been associated with lung cancer, multiple myeloma, and lymphomas, to name a few. Blood tests, bone scans, CAT scans of the chest, abdomen and pelvis, and even bone marrow biopsy can help rule out cancer.

In summary, you should know:

- Is this a peripheral neuropathy?

- Have you ruled out cancer, HIV, or other very dangerous causes?

- Do your tests clearly indicate a particular cause?

- If the tests don't show the cause, are there other tests you need?

- Should you see a neuromuscular or peripheral neuropathy sub-specialist?

- What are the treatments for your neuropathy—first, what are the treatments that might halt the disease, and second, what are the treatments that might reduce symptoms such as pain or fatigue?

There are many treatments for the various peripheral neuropathies. They can be divided into two groups: *disease-modifying treatments* that target the underlying disease, and *symptomatic treatments* that reduce the symptoms but don't alter the course of the underlying disease. I will discuss symptomatic treatments in detail later on.

Disease modifying treatments include medications that lower blood sugar in diabetes, cancer chemotherapy for cancer induced neuropathy, and a variety of treatments for autoimmune neuropathies, including intravenous immunoglobulin, plasma exchange, steroids, and drugs that suppress the immune system such as cytoxan.

John Senneff has written two books on diagnosis and treatment.

In *Numb Toes and Aching Soles* he reviews many kinds of treatment, from disease modifying treatment, to a large number of treatments for pain, and goes on to talk about vitamins, supplements, herbs, experimental, and complementary treatments. In *Numb Toes and Other Woes* he provides an update on pain medications, including newer experimental treatments, and goes on to talk about non-medication treatments such as psychotherapy. Recently published is *The Official Patient's Sourcebook on Peripheral Neuropathy: A Revised and Updated Directory for the Internet Age* (Paperback) by Icon Health Publications, which contains extensive references to the Internet to help you keep up to date on treating your own disease Also consider: *Peripheral Neuropathy: When the Numbness, Weakness, and Pain Won't Stop (American Academy of Neurology)* by Norman Latov MD.

> There are also more technical books and articles that will update you about neuropathy. If you go to the National Library of Medicine on the Internet (www.ncbi.nlm.nih.gov/PubMed/) you can enter search terms such as "diabetic neuropathy" AND "drug treatments') and read abstracts of the latest articles. There is a tutorial program that will teach you how to search for the information you need. Be careful of the remedies you try; Virgil once said: "His sickness increases from the remedies applied to cure it."

Finally, carefully consider the skills and personality of the neurologist you choose. Dismiss any doctor who tells you that there is **nothing** that can be done for you. The online CIDP/ Guillan Barre groups are full of horror stories of people who were told to go home and die, only to seek further advice and get a better outcome. The most any doctor should tell you is that *they* can't think of anything else to do at present. You should ask to be referred to other specialists to see what else might help. It is reasonable for a doctor to say that you have not responded to standard treatments and it might not be worth the risk to try experimental treatment at the present time. It is also important for you to get treatment for the disabilities caused by the illness, such as depression, anxiety, fatigue, weakness, and pain. As I will discuss over and over, it is almost always possible to treat this range of problems and to improve the quality of life of the patient. It is never reasonable for a doctor to take away all hope by giving up on you.

Dismiss as a quack anyone who promises "a complete cure" or 100% success or other similar unrealistic claims. Real treatments have real failure rates. In my illness, CIDP, a 2006 study of 38 patients showed that about a quarter of patients responded very well to a first line treatment, and all but 13% responded at least partially to treatment. People like me, who responded essentially not at all, the "13%ers," need to wait to see how experimental treatments pan out, and to use physical therapy and psychotherapy to maximize our quality of life, although I suspect at this point I am in a poor prognosis group (up the creek without a paddle). As such, I am particularly interested in "complementary and alternative medicine," but these sorts of treatments, especially involving herbs and nutrients, also need to be carefully evaluated. There should be good evidence in the medical literature that at the least a proposed herbal is safe, and some evidence of effectiveness in published studies. A good starting place is the National Center for Complementary and Alternative Medicine (www.nccam.nih.gov).

First I was given intravenous immunoglobulin (IVIG) but on the fourth treatment day my blood pressure went up to 200/ 110, I developed a rash, and the treatment was stopped. Next I had a surgeon place a central line into my heart from a vein in my neck. This was used for a plasma exchange machine (plas-

mapharesis), which takes all the antibodies out of blood and just puts back blood cells mixed with saline or albumin. I felt sick and dizzy with each treatment but the nurses helped me ride it out. No effect. Next was 90 days of high dose prednisone, also with no effect; mercifully without side effect. When this failed I had flunked all three first line treatments for CIDP. Pretty damn bad luck—the disease only affects about 1/ 100,000 people and about 87% of them do respond to a first line treatment. So back to the infusion center at the cancer center for IV cytoxan to suppress my immune system. As I lurched down the hallway to the center with my two arm canes, Chrissie, my nurse, yelled out "run, Forest, run!" The great thing about the infusion center was the constant humor to keep spirits up. The staff didn't defer to me because I was a doctor; rather they treated me, my disease, and everything with a reassuring irreverence. Not to mention that whenever I got a dangerous reaction (super high blood pressure, central line infection, hives from plasma infusion) they were the first responders and they pulled me out of harm's way each time.

II
Dealing with a Diagnosis of Peripheral Neuropathy

Behavioral health specialists look at particular characteristics of your illness to help understand the challenges of coping with the illness (*Psychiatric Care of the Medical Patient, 2nd ed., Stoudemire et. al*). These characteristics include:

- Degree of predictability

- Degree of disability

- Stigma

- Degree of monitoring

- Certainty of prognosis

    Phases you will go through also influence your coping abilities, so you need to be aware of certain phases such as:

- Phase of the illness

- Phase of life

- Phase of your reaction to illness

- Phase of the family's response to illness

The degree of predictability means the ability to predict the course of the illness over time. This is hard to do with many neuropathies, which can be relapsing-remitting or chronic and progressive, leading to chronic feelings of insecurity, feelings of pending doom, even feelings of anxiety during a remission, wondering when "the next shoe will drop." *The way to deal with this is to learn ways to live in the moment—which is very hard to do, even for healthy people.* In an article entitled "Why It's So Hard to Be Happy," by Michael Wiederman (Scientific American Mind February/March 2007, 36-43) the author talks about "going with the flow." Psychologist Mihaly Csikszentmihalyi first coined the term "flow" in 1975 to describe experiences that are not only interesting and motivating but also cause the person to become totally absorbed and fully engaged. Finding activities that produce flow may be crucial to fighting frustration and living in the present. Mindfulness meditation (and many other kinds of meditation and relaxation techniques) combines Western and Eastern philosophies and has proven effective for sufferers of many chronic illnesses. Popularized by Dr. Jon Kabat-Zinn (author of *Full Catastrophe Living*) at the University of Massachusetts Medical School, many hospitals and organizations run stress reduction and mindfulness seminars.

The degree of disability is the extent to which the neuropathy interferes with everyday life. Chronic fatigue is common even when other symptoms such as pain are in remission. The combination of pain, fatigue, and weakness can be overwhelming. *This needs to be dealt with by working with a team that includes physical and occupational therapists, your doctors, your family, and your friends.* I will discuss pain, fatigue, and weakness separately later on.

Stigma results from the negative views of society toward an illness. Stigma associated with neuropathy is minimal since so few people know what neuropathy is. One form of stigma is other people not believing that we have an illness because there are not a lot of obvious signs of illness in many of us. We have what is called "an invisible illness." Sometimes people don't even believe we are ill or deserving of their attention or help. This can be very frustrating when people tell you that "you look so good." This issue is being addressed by Rest Ministries, which sponsors a yearly "National Invisible Chronic Illness Awareness Week" (www.restministries.com or www. invisibleillness.com) in the hopes of bringing help and attention to those of us who look so good but feel so bad. The site www.butyoudontlooksick.com also offers valuable help.

The degree of monitoring is how closely the medical team is likely to watch you. Usually there is intense monitoring and testing during the initial evaluation, which gets less and less intense over time as the diagnosis of neuropathy is made. Sometimes the doctor gets fatigued in caring for the patient and sees the patient less and less often or is less inclined to try new treatments. The patient's response to this must be to insist on regular visits and repeat testing at regular intervals for things that may change. Most importantly, ***work with a primary care physician and neurologist who will respond immediately to any changes or any other illnesses.*** This is **very important**, as any other illnesses, even the flu, may worsen your neuropathy even temporarily, and neuropathy patients get all the same common illnesses other patients get.

The degree of certainty of diagnosis and prognosis (outcome) is low. As many as 25 percent of neuropathy patients will never have the underlying cause found. The prognosis may vary a lot according to the patient. Here, knowledge is your ally. Read about neuropathy, attend support group meetings, and look at studies through the Internet and make sure your doctor's explanation of the diagnosis and treatment make sense. *If it doesn't, get a second opinion. Because of the uncertainty, and the possibility that a negative test will turn positive, discuss with your doctor whether certain tests need to be repeated every year.*

How you cope will also be affected by the *phase of the illness, the phase of life you are in, and the phase of reaction to illness you are in.* **Phase of illness** refers to whether the illness is just diagnosed, acutely active, chronic but stable, chronic but relapsing, or terminal. Your response to illness will be affected by the stage you are in. It is easier to make changes in a chronic illness that is stable than during a relapse. If you are just diagnosed and undergoing treatment, you may need to focus in the here and now and not on future role changes.

Phase of life refers to your life cycle. Are you young and on your own? Are you recently married? Are your kids school age or out of the house? Are you near or in retirement? The problems you face will also be related to your phase of life. You may need to get your children's teachers and guidance counselors to offer them additional support. You may need marriage counseling depending upon how the illness impacts your relationship. You may also need financial counseling to deal with money issues and retirement plans.

Phase of your reaction to illness brings to mind Elizabeth Kubler-Ross' classic stages of dealing with dying, which I think are also useful in looking at dealing with chronic illness. The stages she identifies are denial, anger, bargaining, resignation, and acceptance. If you are still in denial you are unlikely to accept a change in your role. If you are still angry you may resist changing roles

Most of us try to deny our illness at some point. One example of denial is continuing to work or pushing ourselves to maintain our daily schedule despite enormous fatigue. Anger at the disease, and even at doctors is common. Bargaining is common—at each stage of my illness I have said, "if this is as bad as it gets I can live with it, as long as nothing gets worse." There are times when I have a depressed resignation to "my miserable circumstances." Finally, there are times when I accept the illness, aware that I have it, but choose to live in the present, enjoying what I can. Having a chronic illness that causes disability requires a change in coping skills.

Dr. Joann LeMaistre is a psychologist who developed multiple sclerosis. She went on to write a book called *After the Diagnosis* (Alpine Guild, Inc., 1999). An overview of her ideas about coping with chronic illness is on the Internet and quite useful. She also has organized the response to illness in stages:

- crisis

- isolation

- anger

- reconstruction

- intermittent depression

- renewal

During *crisis* you and your family will be very active in fighting the disease and mobilizing resources. Survival of the patient and family is the immediate goal. Most people deal with a crisis reasonably well.

After crisis, *isolation* sets in. There is less attention paid to you by family, friends, and doctors. You may feel that nobody understands the depth of your losses, and stop reaching out to others. In this phase it is important for you to reach out to others.

Next comes *anger*, which may be the most dangerous phase. You can't get angry at fate, and so you may become angry with yourself, even believing you did something bad to deserve the illness. Your family may become angry that you are chronically ill. Even your doctor may be angry that you have failed to get better, despite his or her best efforts.

In this phase suicidal thoughts are common. You need to refocus yourself on goals that you can attain. Suicide is a permanent solution to a temporary problem. How can you call my problem temporary, you ask, if it is incurable? This is because I believe, as does Dr. LeMaistre, that the problem is not the illness but finding self-esteem, value in your life, and new goals, and that this is possible no matter what the disease is.

The last three *phases—reconstruction, intermittent depression, and renewal*—involve attempting to master new coping skills mixed with bouts of depression for what you have lost and working on living in the present. These are subjects we will look at in the remaining chapters of this booklet.

*When I first got sick, I maintained the attitude that as long as all I had to do was walk with a cane and go for treatments to the infusion center on Saturdays the illness "was no big deal." I tried to keep my family (and my boss) calm. I thought I could cope with the crisis just fine; after all, I made my living as a psychiatrist coping with other people's crises. I continued "bargaining with God" over the first few years. With each decline in my health I would say, "if this is the worst it gets I can live with this." Then anger set in—why did **my** life have to get messed up? Isolation also ensued. I dropped out of touch with old friends, and having moved to a new city only two years before I got sick, I wasn't making any new friends. When I saw friends and relatives at parties we didn't know what to say to each other. A lot of people would just pat me on the back and move on after a brief conversation. Others would look down at their shoes. I wasn't much better; I didn't have much skill in being comfortable as a handicapped man. These days, I go back and forth between depression, anger, resignation, and reconstruction. Little by little I learn to cope with my disability. It took me three years in a wheelchair before I got driving lessons to learn to drive with hand controls. It took longer for me to start volunteer work. I am a work in progress, never knowing if I can truly recapture a meaningful life.*

The phase of family stress will differ for each family. Coping with family stress really has two components: how you cope with your family's reaction to your illness and how your family deals with your illness.

"As Gregor Samsa awoke one morning from uneasy dreams he found himself transformed in his bed into a gigantic insect" Thus begins Franz Kafka's well-known novella "The Metamorphosis." The story starts with this premise and follows Samsa and his family trying to deal with this change in their lives. The story fascinates me even more since I began working with chronically ill people. We get illnesses that totally change our sense of ourselves and changes how other people look at us. Like Gregor's family, our significant others can mourn our transition, miss us, and be repelled or overwhelmed by us. In the story, Gregor dies in the end and his family then starts to see a brighter future. I like to think that the families of disabled people can have a happier outcome, but I think the story reveals the ambivalence and pain that others may experience towards us (and the frustration and resentment we may experience towards others) when we are no longer normal, working members of society. Many different interpretations of the story have been made, but common ones deal with society's treatment of those who are different, and the loneliness of being cut off.

Your family may go through similar stages as you, including denial, frustration, and acceptance. This can lead to some difficulties. For example, your spouse may turn to your children or his or her own family of origin to confide in rather than talk openly with you. Family members may feel guilty if they are not constantly with you despite the fact that they need some alone time, and there are things they want to do that you can no longer share with them. Your spouse, children, or significant other may try to take on your role as well as theirs and end up with feelings of martyrdom or resentment. Your family may not openly discuss the illness, fearing that talking about it will only make matters worse, or that upsetting you will make you sicker.

You need to take an active role in discussing these issues with your family and friends. It is important to keep the lines of communication open, and to be direct with your family about what is helpful and what is not.

You may feel jealous or angry with the members of your family who are still healthy. You may feel that they fail to really "understand you." You may feel guilt at what burdens you place on your family. You may feel unwanted even when this is not the case. You may feel panicky at the thought that your family might abandon you. You may blame yourself for any hardships your illness imposes on your family despite the fact that you could not control getting ill. You may resist help in your need to prove your continued independence, or, you may become overly helpless and needy

You and your family will have to deal with the rest of the world. Obvious examples are dealing with employers, financial stressors, and dealing with your medical team. There may be other issues, such as embarrassment about discussing how the illness affects the family with friends and other outsiders. Your illness may affect your children's comfort with their friends and teachers. The stress of the illness may affect their moods. Strongly consider marital and family therapy as well as individual therapy for children stressed out by the changes a chronically ill person brings to a family. You should remember that your illness might magnify pre-existing problems in your marriage and other relationships. There are statistics that indicate a high divorce rate, perhaps more than 75%, in couples where one member gets chronically ill. Early intervention on your part as the ill member of the couple to get extra help and try to keep the relationship healthy is very important.

Jordan, age 12:

"Hello I am here to tell you what life is like growing up with a father that has neuropathy. It is always kind of different. I go outside and see fathers out playing catch or football with their sons. I feel saddened when I see this. I love my dad but he is no Lance Armstrong. Instead unlike most families my dad stays at home while my mom works. Although despite his disease he still manages to be a great father. He helps me when I need help and he is always comforting and loving to me. When I was younger I couldn't understand what was wrong with my dad. I always thought of him like everyone else. He is different but I love him just the same. It was really cool to find out that my dad could drive again. He has this little knob on his car that makes it brake and go. I have a question that all young kids face when their parents have an uncommon disease. The question is, is daddy going to be all right? When I figured it out I was kind of scared. I got over it though. Through my dad's disease I manage to get on. I love my dad and I wouldn't change him for the world."

III
Dealing with Changing Roles

A friend of mine became a paraplegic after an accident. She was a psychiatric resident with me, and she used her illness as a way of teaching her patients. We trained in Philadelphia, which, like most large cities, can be hard to navigate for a disabled person. My friend noted that in the winter the snowplows would pile the snow up on the curbs, making it impossible for her to cross the street alone. She observed that most people would walk by her very quickly, averting their eyes. Once in a while someone would come up behind her, grab the handles of her wheelchair and start pushing, but invariably in *the wrong direction.* She realized that she would have to tell people exactly what she wanted them to do for her and own responsibility for getting the right kind of help. *This capacity to take charge of your illness is critical to dealing with your illness successfully.*

Your chief job is to define a new role for yourself based on what you are now physically and mentally able to do. You may lose your role as a primary breadwinner but be able to take over more household responsibilities or childcare. You may have to change jobs or change your hours. You may have to find new hobbies to replace ones you can no longer participate in. This will take some time and exploration. There will be times you desperately want to go back to your old role, and feel angry and cheated about what has happened to you. Still, many people manage over time to find fulfillment in new roles. *"Happiness is a matter of one's most ordinary everyday mode of consciousness being busy and lively and unconcerned with self. To be damned is for one's ordinary everyday mode of consciousness to be unremitting agonizing preoccupation with self."—Iris Murdoch (b. 1919), British novelist, philosopher.* You cannot afford to simply "become your illness" or to let it consume your thoughts and your time. Furthermore, looking for a new identity is fraught with trying to avoid "all or nothing" thinking. For example: (taken from *The Chronic Illness Experience* by Cheri Register)

- You can tough it out with too little help OR become overly dependent on your doctor and family

- You can keep your illness a secret and avoid thinking about it OR you can discuss it openly and become self-pitying

- You can ask for help and risk being a burden OR be too independent and isolate yourself

- You can push yourself to the limit and risk getting sicker OR you can do too little and be more of an invalid than necessary

- You can be angry about your illness and then bitter OR you can focus only on counting your blessings and risk being self-delusional

The search for a happy medium is something each sufferer must go through to find an identity while managing the effects of the illness.

Debbie Dawson RN is both a nurse and fellow peripheral neuropathy sufferer. She has written on how she divides her roles and activities into five "compartments." (From Debbie Dawson, RN, who suffers from CIDP, leader of Delaware County Neuropathy Support Group)

1. Things I can no longer do (for example, power walking).

2. Things I couldn't do before, but can now (have time to write and do crafts).

3. Things I do the same as before (like sitting in the sunroom watching a sunset).

4. Things I can still do, but differently (can go to a mall, but need a wheelchair).

5. Things I can do differently, just not ready to yet (such as go to a Phillies game)

This is a very clever way to help examine your life and get going on things you wish to do. I have been talking with Debbie about my wish to take my family on a cruise, and she wrote back: "Remember the five categories—you can do them all in one shot! Here's a chance to turn a 1 (can't do), into a 5 (not ready to do), then into a 4 (do, but differently than you would have before). And on the side you do a 2 (wouldn't have had the time to do before), and throw in a lot of 3's (watching those sunsets, indulging in the cruise pampering, laughing with your family). These will be the same, chair or not! Go for it!"

I have been unable to practice psychiatry for several years as of this writing. I am just beginning to develop new roles and interests. So don't punish yourself if it takes a long time to come to terms with the changes in your life.

Here are some ideas for dealing with your changing roles:

1. *Ask yourself exactly what it was about your previous job or activities that was most enjoyable.* For a long time I just said that I couldn't stand how much I missed being a psychiatrist. With the help of my therapist I was able to see that helping people and teaching were the parts of my work that I enjoyed the most. So while I can't maintain a regular practice, there are plenty of ways to help others, and opportunities for me to volunteer to teach.

2. *Talk with a specialist.* You can contact your local Office of Vocational Rehabilitation. You can have your doctor give you a prescription to see an occupational therapist. The occupational therapist can work with you on adaptive equipment, ways to conserve energy, and other techniques that permit you to do more even with a disability. There are also psychologists and therapists who specialize in vocational counseling.

3. *Stop beating up on yourself.* You did not get sick because "unconsciously" you were lazy and didn't want to work anymore. Peripheral neuropathy is a serious illness and you have to give yourself credit for whatever you manage to accomplish.

4. *Organize your goals, and set small goals you can meet.* For example my goal last year was to keep going to physical therapy, not let myself quit, and be able to walk for ½ hour at a time. My physical therapist helped me keep the goal small—if I had aimed higher I would have failed, and probably quit trying.

5. *Try something new.* Just try it—you are under no obligation to like it. I was in the hospital and given a crafts project to do to pass the time. Normally I don't do crafts and I thought that I didn't like that sort of thing. But I did enjoy this project, and to my own surprise, I bought some crafts equipment when I got home.

6. *If you stay employed know your rights.* Make sure you know your rights under the Americans with Disabilities Act (ADA) as well as Family and Medical Leave Act (FMLA). It is reasonable to negotiate for accommodations, both physical ones as well as time flexibility accommodations. The Job Accommodations Network provides individualized counsel for disabled individuals and a great deal of information including self-employment options at http://www.jan.wvu.edu or **800-526-7234.**

You may ask yourself: how can I ever be happy again? Changing roles may have a profound impact on your identity, and for some people (possibly for men more than women) career is closely associated with self-worth. I might ask how happy you really were to begin with if you really have such low self-esteem from changes in your roles.

Brenda was a 30-year old woman with a 15-year history of bipolar (manic-depressive) disorder. She had been stable for several years on lithium and haldol and she saw me every 3 months in the outpatient clinic for "a med check." During the first five minutes of her 20 minute session we would review her medication use, effects, side effects, lab tests and so on. I was a second year resident reading about bipolar disorder in textbooks; she had lived with it for fifteen years. She knew way more about managing her disease than I did. After the five minutes of medication review she would tell me about her everyday life. She worked as a cashier at the local K-Mart. After work she went to a gym with friends. She went out frequently with friends and lived with her family with whom she got along well. She helped her sick mother out at home but even with this she had a lot of time to pursue her own interests. She was happy, well adjusted, and content with her situation and enjoyed life.

At the time I "picked up" Brenda in my caseload I was a second year resident with long hours, frequent overnight on-call duty at the hospital, and little free time. I began to consider the meaning of "the K-Mart effect" where I consistently saw people with less education than me and perhaps more limited career goals far outstripping me in personal happiness. I spent high school preparing for college, college preparing for med school, med school preparing for residency, and residency preparing for a life of practice that would require continuous educational updates and recertifications. At every step I was coached to achieve more, get higher grades, and work harder. Approval was hard to win and every "A" only meant the potential humiliation of slipping and suffering the humiliation of a B. My first paid hospital job was to work as a janitor at a local hospital. Even then I noticed my tendency to feel pressured to get my work done well, while the experienced janitors focused on pacing themselves to a relaxing day in which the job was done and they went home without exhaustion.

Clearly, happiness hinges upon a great deal more (and less) than your job title. The "positive psychology" literature I mentioned earlier on why it's hard to be happy is growing and psychologists are working on better, more scientific studies on how to achieve happiness. How can *you* achieve happiness in the face of a life-altering disease? I don't know. I only know from my experience as a therapist that it is possible. The process of redefining and rebuilding is unique for every person. I have made a lot of mistakes in therapy with chronically ill/disabled persons; usually based on underestimating the emotional cost of accepting a change in the patient's life. Now, working from a wheelchair, I understand better. Sometimes a chronically ill person just "doesn't wanna" accept a change, even if intellectually they admit it might improve their life. Healthy, fully abled people have a right to not do things just because they don't feel like it; why should it be different for the chronically ill?

Moreover, the are some important lessons from the study of happiness (USA Today 12/8/2002 online edition):

- Good health is not a prerequisite for happiness; researchers found happy ill people and unhappy healthy people
- About half your tendency to be happy is genetic and unrelated to your life circumstances
- Happy people pursue personal growth; they tend not to measure themselves against the achievement of others
- Satisfaction comes most often when engaged in "flow" activities (previously discussed) that are absorbing and keep the person focused in the present.

- Everyone has some special strengths which can be called into use and allow them to handle a difficult situation in their own unique way
- Gratitude helps—expressing what you are grateful for improves happiness
- Forgiveness is closely linked with happiness
- Altruistic acts—volunteering to help others—strongly helps with personal happiness
- People are built to be resilient, to bounce back more quickly then they would expect from a bad situation

There are websites, discussion groups, and message boards for different types of neuropathy on the Internet. Start with The Neuropathy Association's websites: www.neuropathy.org and www.neuropathy.com.

Also try http://www.compassnet.com/winoverpn for a website with lots of coping tips. The various peripheral neuropathy chat groups and websites change address so you should search the internet for "peripheral neuropathy," "peripheral neuropathy support groups" and so on, including doing a Google search of your specific disease by name. Yahoo and other portals also have lists of online groups you can look up. You should also attempt to find a local support group or communicate by mail, phone, or Internet with fellow sufferers. Talk to fellow sufferers—they have the best firsthand knowledge and have learned the most novel ways to cope—because they have to.

The first few years after I had to stop working I had no interest in doing anything else. After all, being a psychiatrist 24/7 had been my life, and I enjoyed it so much that I did it as a hobby too, bring-

ing home stacks of journals to pour over every night, getting on my computer at three in the morning to search for more options for patients of mine. At least I had the online message groups. I became friends with fellow sufferers from all over the world. I got messages from New Zealand, England, and Israel. Lots of tips and hints but mostly mutual encouragement.

I took my new role as "stay at home Dad" pretty tough. I love my kids but taking care of three kids all day is much rougher than treating an entire emergency room full of suicidally depressed patients. Psychiatry is something I felt mastery of but being a good psychiatrist has absolutely no impact on being a good parent or for that matter husband. My wife has stayed encouraging and supportive throughout our ordeal and with her help I gradually learned my kids' names and birth dates, when they had band and after school activities, and what school papers had to be signed.

IV
Dealing with an Emotional Crash

Do you ever have a day when you feel that everything you do is hard? You have trouble concentrating, you feel keyed up; everything you do makes you tenser. You feel more irritable, easily upset, and out of control. Everything you have to do seems terribly important, and you can't decide what to do first. Your problems seem insurmountable and you can't see any way out.

If you feel this way, rush to your phone and call 1-800-BUY-CRAP and for only $19.99 I will mail you a one-month supply of Dr. Scott's Stress-Free Pills. This amazing new formula is so potent it can make your children behave better, give you a better sex life, get a raise at work, and help you lose 20, 30, or even 50 dollars to me in just 4 weeks!! You can also call a psychic, get advice in Internet chat rooms, buy the latest edition of a women's or men's magazine, pray, meditate, ask your family doctor for tranquilizers, use street drugs, drink heavily, beat somebody up, or sell your soul to Satan. I doubt, however, that any of these options will make you feel much better. Even the healthier ones, like prayer and meditation probably won't help because if they did help, you wouldn't be feeling like this. If you are feeling overwhelmed:

1. **Admit that your judgment is shot**. This is critical. As long as you hold on to having to be in control and believing that your view of the world is the only view you won't feel better. Don't be embarrassed; there are times when everyone loses his or her judgment. I asked a senior therapist once whether everyone feels suicidal at some time and he replied that everyone has known desperation.

2. **Don't just do something, stand there**. This is the opposite of the old adage as you're used to hearing it, but a standard clinical pearl in psychiatry. If you don't know what to do, stop and take stock, don't just flail about helplessly, trying everything in site, exhausting yourself. This is like a swimmer in distress who starts to drown because he struggles into exhaustion.

3. **Don't try things that have already failed**. This includes alcohol, tobacco, other drugs, staying in bed, or even healthy habits that didn't work for you in the past.

4. **Get help**. Don't just "seek it." Seeking can be rather passive and rather confusing. Call your doctor and ask to be referred to a psychiatrist or psychologist on an urgent basis. Do not accept a one-month delay to be seen; many therapists have some capacity to handle emergencies. In a pinch, go to the nearest emergency room of a hospital that has psychiatric services and a psychiatric unit. Even if you clearly don't want to be admitted, these hospitals have more trained staff to see you in the emergency room; and the ER crisis worker may be able to get you into an outpatient therapist's office in several days.

5. **Be careful about whom you seek counsel from**. Advice that is free is worth every penny, and plenty of people will want to offer you advice. The advice needs to come from someone who you have reason to believe will offer it in the spirit of your best interest and not because of any gain they might get from it. Advice from a parent, spouse, boss and so on might not be your best choice in a crisis. Someone who has positive feelings for you and wants to help you but has nothing to gain or lose by what you do is ideal.

   Let me illustrate. If someone were to come up to you and tell you that your hair or your clothing looked awful you would rightfully be insulted. Yet almost everyone has some friend or confidante who can tell them the same thing and you feel glad they noticed before other people did so you could fix your hair or your clothing. This person is someone you trust, and someone you know is giving advice selflessly. This is the sort of person to talk with when you feel overwhelmed. If you don't know someone like this, find a good therapist. A therapist can be close but objective, caring but not controlling, and recognize when to give advice and when to let you work on a problem yourself.

6. **Make a short term plan and stick with it.** If you seek counsel, make a commitment to following through on what is suggested.

   Often, you will feel that you just can't make a change, or that the timing is wrong, or that a change would be risky. A friend of mine, who is a phenomenal social worker, tells her patients that "the thinking that got you into this problem will never get you out." Often I will be very directive when seeing an overwhelmed patient. This is because being over-whelmed causes enough confusion that it would be hard for the patient to organize his thoughts if I gave him too many options. I'll say things like: "it looks like you're burned out. You can't work, you can't sleep and you see no future. I'm going to put you in the hospital for a few days to give you around the clock care, and when you're feeling calmer we'll pick up with outpatient therapy." Or, "work is too much for you now. You could lose your job if your performance is poor, and you feel miserable going to work. Your concentra-tion is bad, and your depression is severe. This is a perfectly legitimate reason for a medical leave of absence. I'll write you a note and I want you to call out sick. Then talk with your human relations department about what other docu-mentation they need from me. If you need to apply for short-term disability, send me the doctor's statement. I'll see you weekly until you feel better, and I want you to call me if you feel worse."

"Bill" was a 30 year old man who tragically witnessed his 9 year old son being killed by a hit and run driver. He became depressed and suicidal. After several hospitalizations his mood improved to the point that he could get through the day, but he still felt chronically hopeless and helpless. I saw him several weeks before Christmas.

Bill: Well I guess the holidays will really suck this year.

Me: How would you like to spend the Christmas vacation?

Bill: Well I'll spend Christmas Eve with my family. Christ-mas Day I'll visit my in-laws, and then I'll go to my brother's house for dinner. It will be tough, seeing all my nieces and nephews.

Me: How would you *like* to spend the holiday?

Bill: Well I haven't got much choice.

Me: Suppose for a moment that you could do anything you wanted for Christmas, that money, time, distances were all no problem.

Bill: (smiling) I'd get on a plane, fly to Vegas, and try to forget about everything.

Me: So go to Vegas.

Bill: I can't imagine that.

Me: You have already experienced the unimaginable on the bad side of things, so you should let yourself have the unimaginable on the good side.

Bill: I don't know ... I don't want to disappoint my family.

Me: Well try to do something for yourself over the holiday. I'll see you in January.

Bill came back in January; he had convinced his brother to travel with him and spent Christmas week in Vegas, thoroughly enjoying himself.

7. **Establish a medium range plan.** Decide what changes you'll make in the days just after an absence from work, or after a hospitalization. Figure out your daily schedule and make it realistic, tending toward being cautious and doing less than your maximum

8. **Establish a long-range plan.** Decide, with the help of your doctor or therapist, what you need to do to continue to feel more relaxed. If this includes relaxation exercises, going to the gym, dieting, psychotherapy, medication, start it and stick with it. For most psychiatric medicines, "the dose that gets you there is the dose that keeps you there." That is, when you find an effective dose of an antidepressant, mood stabilizer, or anti-anxiety medication, you need to stay on it. Stopping prematurely leads to a large number of relapses, and cutting down to a "maintenance" dose is not as effective as the full dose.

9. **Follow through with the plan.** If I tell you to take a week off, don't go back to work in two days just because you feel a little better. You'll be back in the hole in no time.

10. **Take the help that is offered and ask for help when you need it.** A massive rainstorm causes a small town to flood. Evacuation boats are sent out. The boat stops at the house of the only preacher in town. The preacher refuses to get in the boat, saying, "God will protect me." The next day the preacher is on the second floor of his house, the first floor being flooded. A second boat comes by and the rescuers plead with the preacher to get on board. "God will save me," says the preacher, "I have always been his devoted servant." The next day a third boat comes by to find the preacher stranded on his roof. The rescuers tell him this is the last boat out of town. Again he refuses, certain that God will intervene. The floodwaters rise further and the preacher drowns. He gets to heaven, is welcomed by St. Peter, and goes through the gates to talk to God. "God" he asks, "why

did you forsake me in my time of need?" "What are you talking about," says God, "I sent three boats!"

Whatever support groups are available, whatever agencies provide help, whatever your friends and family offer to do, take the help. You need it, and they are happy to give it. They are your rescue boats. I do not speak from the cheap seats on this one. I have helped many people. As my neurological disease has progressed, I have been glad to have the help of my neurologist, my psychiatrist and psychologist, a visiting nurse and social workers, and many others who have been giving. I don't feel demeaned by this. It would be hypocritical if I did, suggesting that I feel it is all right for my patients, who are lesser in some way, to take help, but I am too good to take help. Taking help feels good as does giving help. Don't reject what you need, and you may be in a position to help someone else someday.

V

Dealing with Weakness and Loss of Coordination

The primary symptoms of peripheral neuropathy are weakness and pain, along with which we group loss of coordination and loss of sensation. Muscle weaknesses accompanying your neuropathy and weakness from not using the muscles in the affected limbs are common. Besides weakness, you may experience difficulty with your balance. This is really a sensory problem, but since it affects your walking I will deal with it in this section. You have several different kinds of nerves in your limbs, and different tracts in the spinal cord that carry different information. Specifically, you have nerves that give your brain information about proprioception, or where your arms and legs are and how they are positioned. Without this information it is hard to coordinate and hard to stand up.

We have three sets of mechanisms that help us stay steady on our feet: the nerves that carry position sense to the dorsal tracts of the spinal cord; our eyes; and the semicircular canals in the inner ear. If the nerves that carry position sense are damaged, we depend on our eyes more. That is why, whenever I go to a neuropathy conference, someone will ask: "how many of you fall over in the dark?" and many people will raise their hands. If your feet can't tell your brain where you are and your eyes can't see, then you will fall. Using nightlights all the time can help. Using a cane, or a pair of canes with arm braces, sends information about the floor to your arms and from there to your brain. In one study of diabetics with neuropathy, it was shown that just being able to touch surfaces lightly with their hands improved their balance. Use whatever combination of walkers, canes, grab bars in showers, shower seats, etc. you need to prevent a fall. Also get a Personal Emergency Response System if you live alone. This is the "I've fallen and I can't get up" button you wear on a bracelet or necklace even in the shower to summon help. The American Red Cross has a program as do a number of private companies. It is wise to get an assessment from a physical therapist to help plan ways to avoid falls. Remember, a fall can set you back or send you to the hospital!

There are a number of useful ways to deal with weakness and loss of coordination. First, find a physical therapist that has experience dealing with chronic diseases. I have found that many physical therapists are more comfortable dealing with injuries in which return to full function is a goal. They work me too hard, set unrealistic goals, and fatigue me so much that I quit the therapy. Physical therapy for the neuropathy patient should be at a slow steady pace, and should not leave you in pain after each session. Your disease is chronic and incurable, so what's the hurry to make progress in physical therapy?

Good occupational therapists can help you in a number of ways. If your hands are affected, they can train you to use your hands more effectively. They can engage you in a program called "work hardening," in which you simulate with them what you do at work and they show you safer, easier ways to do your job. Finally, they are an invaluable resource in buying adaptive equipment (special kitchen utensils, reaching instruments, and so forth) to make life easier. In fact, they can do home visits to evaluate the safety of your home for you, and work with you in "energy saving" techniques where you learn to do familiar tasks in simpler ways or with adaptive equipment so as to save energy for more pleasurable activities.

Finally, you need to take the help and not resist it. One patient of mine kept telling me that using a cane was "giving in to the illness and just a crutch." I asked her to tell me the definition of a crutch.

"Well," she said, "it's something you use to walk with when you break a leg." "Exactly!" I said, "A crutch takes someone who would be confined to a chair and makes them mobile—what's wrong with that?" She went on to get a cane and was very happy with her increased ability to walk.

I had to do a lot of adapting when the nerves in my legs that affect position sense got damaged. First a cane, then a walker, then bilateral arm crutches for short hops and a wheelchair for longer outings. An electric wheelchair for my office and the hospital so I could conserve energy for seeing patients, and hand controls to drive my car. My bathroom has four grab bars so I can hold on in the shower, getting out of the shower, and getting on the toilet. If I close my eyes I hold on to the bars for dear life since I fall even in dim light.

We have nightlights in our bedroom, bathroom, and living room so I can move about at night without falling.

VI
Dealing with Pain and Loss of Sensation

Neuropathy can be extremely painful. The *New England Journal of Medicine* devoted an entire article to "Painful Sensory Neuropathy" (NEJM 348:13, March 27, 2003). The article reviewed over sixteen types of painful neuropathy and the research about treatment. The pain is caused by damage to small nerve fibers, is often debilitating, and responds poorly to treatment.

Let me review some of the treatment for neuropathy pain. First let's look at the difference between pain caused by a wound or an illness and neuropathic pain. Pain caused by a wound is temporary and is important in alerting us to the fact that there is a wound. Pain caused by neuropathy is caused by damage to the nerves even though the surrounding tissues may be perfectly normal, and has no benefit to us. Therefore, neuropathic pain can be looked upon as a disease with underlying causes such as diabetes, injury, toxins, and cancer. Diabetic neuropathy and post-herpetic neuralgia are the leading causes of neuropathic pain. For a detailed explanation, see Gareth Parry, MD, *Neuropathic Pain Treatment: Pathophysiology to Next Gen-*

eration Therapeutics, web lecture at www.medscape.com Neuropathic pain is harder to treat, but every year the treatments get better. Treatments for neuropathic pain include a number of medications:

1. Tricyclic antidepressants such as amitriptyline (Elavil), nortriptyline (Pamelor), desipramine (Norpramin)

2. Other antidepressants such as bupropion (Wellbutrin), venlafaxine (Effexor) and duloxetine (Cymbalta).

3. Anticonvulsants such as gabapentin (Neurontin), pregabalin (Lyrica), oxcarbazepine (Trileptal), carbamazepine (Tegretol), lamotragine (Lamictal), and topiramate (Topomax).

4. Mexiletine (a cardiac drug like lidocaine)

5. Narcotics and narcotic like drugs (Ultram, morphine, oxycodone, hydrocodone)

6. Local anesthetics like topical lidocaine, capsaicin and mixes of medications turned into creams by compounding pharmacists. These creams may contain amitriptyline, ketamine, non-steroidals (ketoprofen), baclofen and other ingredients although their effectiveness is questionable and varies a lot from patient to patient

7. Alternative therapies such as magnets, electrical stimulation.

   Frequently used painkillers such as non-steroidal anti-inflammatory drugs like ibuprofen (Motrin) and COX-2 inhibitors are probably not a good choice for neuropathic pain; similarly SSRIs (like Prozac) are not particularly useful for pain. As of this writing (2007) there are about 100 new drugs in development for pain, almost 30 specifically for neuropathic pain. There is no reason to give up looking for adequate pain control. Careful trials of several meds, combinations of treatments, and treatment combined with non-pharmacological methods (such as meditation) all offer hope.

Pain specialists are doctors who specialize in the treatment of chronic pain in patients who are not likely to get better. They may be helpful to you. You should understand some current concepts of pain medicine:

- Chronic non-malignant (not cancer) pain should be treated aggressively. This is in contrast to a past history of reserving potent narcotics mostly for dying cancer patients.

- Pain is best treated in a multidisciplinary manner with medication, physical therapy, and psychological counseling.

- Pain medication should be monitored carefully.

- Pain medications are often added in "layers," that is, a tricyclic antidepressant may be started and then an anticonvulsant added and later on a narcotic. A long-acting narcotic is often a better choice for chronic, around the clock pain

- Chronic severe pain that is not treated is poor medical care.

Finally, be careful to monitor for loss of sensation. Diabetics often have this problem with their feet, and get sores and infections more easily. Inspect your affected hands or feet regularly. Keep nails trimmed. Make sure that footwear doesn't rub or chafe. Set the temperature on your water heater to 120 degrees to avoid burning numb skin. Occupational therapists can help with safety issues. If your feet are affected, it may be a good idea to have a podiatrist help with foot care.

VII
Dealing with Depression and Anxiety

People are going to tell you that being depressed and anxious is perfectly normal for someone with a chronic painful illness. I agree that this is a normal response. However, it is often expected that since there is a "good reason" for your anxiety and depression you should just put up with it. This is where I disagree. If someone shot you in the chest it would be perfectly normal for you to bleed. However, no one would think of just letting you keep on bleeding. Yet somehow there is a social expectation that you should just put up with anxiety and depression. This is worsened by the continuing stigma regarding treating psychiatric illness. I think this is a pity, because as a psychiatrist I often see the most dramatic responses to treatment in medically ill patients who develop anxiety and depression. The cause of the distress is clear to the patient, the issues of dealing with illness are common across many chronic illnesses, and it is perfectly realistic to see someone continue to have the primary chronic illness but have their anxiety and depression lift considerably. There are lots of good studies documenting effective treatment of depression in all kinds of illness, including cancer and AIDs. Bottom line: insist that your depression be treated vigorously, both with medication and psychotherapy.

Why is treating depression often ignored? There are a number of reasons.

- The patient is unaware that he or she suffers from depression.

- The patient is embarrassed to ask for help.

- The physician fails to make the diagnosis.

- The physician fails to treat the depression, or under-treats it.

- The patient is embarrassed to go to a psychiatrist.

- The patient's doctor or family is embarrassed to talk about psychiatric care with the patient.

- The patient is afraid that the doctors think their neurological symptoms are "all in their head."

Psychiatrists have terms for illnesses that are essentially psychological but show up with lots of physical complaints: "somatoform disorder" "somatoform pain disorder," and "hypochondriasis." I have worked with lots of patients who have been labeled "head cases" by other doctors and I have learned a lot. First, my own illness convinces me that someone can be essentially mentally healthy, get stricken with a chronic and incurable illness, and then develop an incredibly long and unbelievable story (except to fellow sufferers) about their illness. I am frankly skeptical about "psychological" pain disorders. The many patients in whom I have uncovered underlying other medical problems have been very high.

A thirty five year old woman with chronic depression came to see me; she had multiple physical complaints that included joint pain, stomach pain, and rapid heartbeat.

I enlisted the help of several specialists at the hospital, telling them although she was depressed, I did not think it accounted for her physical symptoms. Over two years of investigation she was diagnosed with active rheumatoid arthritis, a heart rhythm disorder, and a rare compression of the artery that feeds the stomach. Each was treated medically or surgically, and her physical symptoms got better.

If you see a psychiatrist or therapist it will be to deal with the emotional issues surrounding your neuropathy. I tell my patients something like this:

"You have some medical illnesses—specifically peripheral neuropathy. These illnesses in and of themselves may not cause depression, but the rate of depression in chronically physically ill patients is much higher than in a healthy population. Besides these illnesses, you have developed poor sleep, poor appetite, low energy, little enjoyment in activities, feelings of worthlessness, feelings of hopelessness, crying spells, and thoughts of death. All together this qualifies you for a diagnosis of depression. If we treat the depression you are going to feel better and you may better be able to fight the other illnesses. But your illnesses are not imaginary or a result of depression. If you respond to antidepressant treatment you will still have neuropathy. While I'm treating you I still want to hear about any new physical symptoms you have so I can think about whether they are a side effect of the treatment or are a matter of concern that I need to call your neurologist about."

One of the most important roles a psychiatrist has as a medical doctor involved in the treatment of mental illnesses is to maintain diagnostic skills about coexisting medical illnesses. Over my years as a consultant, I have been called to see a patient who seemed "anxious" and when I noted her rapid breathing, I did tests that led to a diagnosis of a pulmonary embolus. I have picked up serious GI bleed in a patient who complained of dizziness (from all the fluid he lost), and I have seen multiple "medical" causes of psychosis including low blood sugar, high calcium in a cancer patient, drug withdrawal, low blood pressure, infection, and overdose. A psychiatrist who treats every patient seriously is the last line of defense for patients with unusual symptoms in the general hospital setting.

Treating Depression

Depression is treatable in the face of virtually every known physical disease, including cancer and AIDs. So you should expect to be able to have your depression treated with good responses.

The best treatment for depression is a combination of psychotherapy and medication. Some people prefer therapy or counseling without medication because they already feel overmedicated. Other people feel so bad they can't even talk in therapy and do better when started on medication.

Depression is a serious illness in and of itself. It is one of the leading causes of disability throughout the world, and a one of the most disabling illnesses (not just mental illnesses)—it is a top cause of disability and lost work time up there with cardiac disease, diabetes, and others.

The diagnosis is made when the patient has two weeks or more of depressed mood or loss of pleasure in previously enjoyable activities, along with five of the following symptoms. These are sleep changes, low interest, feelings of guilt or worthlessness, low energy, poor concentration, changes in appetite, and suicidal thoughts. It can be a Major Depressive episode by these criteria. It can also be a depressed phase of Bipolar (manic-depressive) Disorder: most manic—depressives spend a lot more time depressed than in manic phase. The depression can also have psychotic features, such as delusions or hallucinations. A psychiatric examination is usually sufficient to make the diagnosis; standardized tests such as the Beck Depression Inventory can help document the presence, symptoms, and severity of depression. Medical tests can look for co-existing conditions that can contribute to depression (e.g. hypothyroidism, anemia).

There are many good antidepressants, with more coming out each year. We used to group them into categories, but there are too many to group at this point.

The first line antidepressants are the Selective Serotonin Reuptake Inhibitors (SSRIs), which include fluoxetine (Prozac), sertraline (Zoloft), fluvoxamine (Luvox), paroxetine (Paxil), citalopram (Celexa), and escitalopram (Lexapro). While not terribly good for pain, they are reliable antidepressants with good safety profiles. I often choose Celexa or Lexapro for my medically ill patients as they have very few interactions with other drugs. Tricyclic antidepressants such as amitriptyline (Elavil), nortriptyline (Pamelor) or imipramine (Tofranil) do have some effect on pain as well as depression but have more side effects. Newer antidepressants include mirtazepine (Remeron), bupropion (Wellbutrin), venlafaxine (Effexor), and nefazadone (Serzone). Wellbutrin may also help pain. Effexor can treat both depression and anxiety and possibly can reduce pain. Duloxetine (Cymbalta) is most recently released and is effective for both depression and diabetic neuropathy pain. Serzone and Remeron can be sedating and help with sleep. St. John's Wort is only partially effective and only for mild depression. Psychostimulants may help with depression and fatigue; these include Ritalin, Dexedrine, and Provigil (modafenil).

Depression can be tough to treat, and the chances of a full remission on any one antidepressant are probably less than 60 %. Good treatment involves an adequate dose for a reasonable length of time (2-6 weeks), and careful selection of a second drug if the first one doesn't work. A full treatment course may require one or two medication switches, adding "boosting" agents such as lithium, thyroid hormone, buspar, and others, or using two antidepressants at once. For resistant depression ECT (electroconvulsive therapy) can be safe, rapid acting, and importantly, safe in physically ill patients.

There are many kinds of psychotherapy, but only a small number have the research to back up that they work. Interpersonal therapy looks at the interaction of the depression with key life problems such as grief, difficulty in coping with new roles and role changes. So we can see how this kind of therapy might lend itself to work with medically ill patients who are mourning the loss of their health, and trying to cope with new and less familiar roles. Cognitive-behavior psychotherapy helps you to correct "distorted" thinking such as thinking "everything is going wrong" when only one thing is going wrong. Make sure your therapist has training in therapy techniques in one or more of the currently used therapies.

Overall, there is good reason to be hopeful about recovering from depression even in the face of a chronic physical illness that is not curable. I have seen many patients with neuropathic pain, chronic lung disease, cancer, and other chronic illnesses brighten up considerably with proper psychiatric care. As an added benefit, I think that chronic illness stays better controlled in patients in whom depression is adequately treated.

The "old goal" of antidepressant treatment was a "response" to the medication, usually considered a 50% remission in depression score on a standard scale. However, 50% of miserable is still pretty rotten, and patients who got a response without a full remission had residual symptoms, didn't do as well as full responders, and relapsed more often. Now the initial goal is to put the depression into remission (achieve a normal score on a standardized depression scale). Although this is much harder to achieve it is indicative of overall better treatments now and in the near future that we can aim higher.

Treating Anxiety

Anxiety is to be expected in the face of being diagnosed with a chronic illness. Anxiety can take many forms. It may be specific worries about the illness such as:

- Fear of relapse or worsening

- Fear of disability

- Fear of isolation

- Fear of stigma

- Fear of pain

   The anxiety may present itself as constant worry, tension, or inability to concentrate, known as Generalized Anxiety Disorder. Some patients experience panic attacks, sudden bouts of severe terror with shortness of breath, pounding heart, and a feeling of fright that something awful is about to happen. A social anxiety with fear of going out in public may occur as you see yourself differently with the disease.

There is no reason to suffer from chronic anxiety. There are very good treatments, including:

- Psychotherapy, including cognitive-behavioral therapy (CBT): CBT involves learning to recognize the negative thoughts that lead to anxious feelings. Behavior therapy can include relaxation technique, gradual exposure to feared situations, and other techniques that allow mastery of fearful situations.

- Relaxation training, which includes breathing exercises and progressive muscle relaxation

- Spiritual and faith based help

- Non-medication methods such as exercise and massage

- Medication treatment

There are a wide variety of medications that help with anxiety. Although some of them can be habit forming, I have observed that very few patients with true anxiety disorders abuse their medication. Medications fall into several categories:

Benzodiazepines. These include diazepam (Valium), chlordiazepoxide (Librium), alprazolam (Xanax), lorazepam (Ativan), clonazepam (Klonopin) and others. Although they are controlled drugs, which can be habit forming, they have the advantages of being highly effective and very safe, as well as working very quickly.

Antidepressants. A number of antidepressants have been shown to be effective in treating anxiety even in non-depressed patients. These include Paxil, Lexapro, Zoloft, and Effexor. Duloxetine (Cymbalta) will possibly be effective. Remeron helps sleep and anxiety, and Serzone has a modest anti-anxiety effect. The older tricyclics, such as Elavil and imipramine, are useful for some forms of anxiety. Clomipramine works for obsessive-compulsive disorder and panic attacks. You should be aware that antidepressants given for anxiety take several weeks of daily dosing to work; no single dose will stop an anxiety attack. Sometimes a benzodiazepine is given for a short time until the antidepressant starts to work.

Antipsychotics. Although most neuropathy patients don't have psychotic symptoms (like hearing voices or having delusional beliefs), the new "atypical antipsychotics" have been noted by many psychiatrists to have anti-anxiety properties. Quetiapine (Seroquel), risperidone (Risperdal), and olanzapine (Zyprexa) in particular may help with anxiety that doesn't respond to other medications. Although these drugs may have side effects, they are well tolerated at the lower doses used for anxiety and are not habit forming

Others. Gabapentin (Neurontin) and pregabalin (Lyrica) may have anti-anxiety effects. Hydroxyzine (Atarax,Vistaril) is an antihistamine with proven anti-anxiety effects. Some herbal medications such as valarian may help, but be careful. Herbal medications in large doses are drugs, and have side effects. For example, kava-kava was taken off the shelves in Europe because it caused liver damage, and tryptophan was taken off the shelf in the U.S. because of a dangerous reaction called eosino-philia—myalgia syndrome.

I have had significant anxiety and depression as a result of my illness. Antidepressants and antianxiety medication have helped control symptoms. Just as important, psychotherapy has helped me to adapt. I have fewer fantasies that I will ever get better and I invest more of myself in my children and in writing and volunteer work. I can contemplate the possibility of never practicing psychiatry again without totally freaking out, even though it fills me with deep sadness. Dealing with reality and still trying to be responsible for what happens to me is a process. It's easy to see myself as a victim and then take a helpless role. I don't think I could have made it through this ordeal without this help. And when I overdo it, my doctors are there to help and to be firm with me that I respect my limits.

VIII
Dealing with Fatigue and Insomnia

I will deal with these topics together because they often go hand in hand, and many neuropathy patients will have both at some time. Insomnia can cause fatigue, as can the medicines used to treat insomnia. Fatigue and pain can worsen insomnia.

Fatigue is a fact of life for many neuropathy patients. Often our families and friends fail to appreciate this because "we look so good." In fact, in one study looking at fatigue in autoimmune neuropathy (*"Fatigue in Immune-Mediated Polyneuropathies," Neurology* 53: 8 November 1999, I.S.J. Merkies, et al) 80 percent of 113 patients had severe fatigue. The fatigue was independent of motor or sensory symptoms, and was rated as one of the top three most disabling symptoms.

There are some treatments for fatigue. First, treatment that targets the underlying disease, such as insulin for diabetes, or IVIG for autoimmune neuropathy, may help the fatigue. Other medications, such as stimulants (Ritalin, Provigil) may help. In fact, Provigil, a new agent that promotes wakefulness, has been effective in open trials in a number of chronic illnesses. Amantadine and acetylcarnitine have been used in trials with multiple sclerosis, but thus far there have been no other specific anti-fatigue drugs commercially available. Non-pharmacologic approaches such as exercise, relaxation training, and physical therapy may be helpful. In particular, therapy in a warm pool may be useful and put less stress on joints.

Learning to conserve energy is helpful and important. An occupational therapist may be able to work with you and even do a home visit to help you organize things and get adaptive equipment. The goal is to use less energy to get basic chores done so that you have more energy for other activities. Along the same lines, getting help from others in house cleaning, marketing, and so forth may be necessary, even though it is difficult for some people to ask. You will probably develop some personal ways to fight fatigue.

In my family room I have a big comfortable recliner to rest and nap in. The phone, the TV remote control, my laptop computer, a magazine rack, and a small plastic filing box are all within reach without my getting out of my "nappy chair." I prefer to use this chair even when I am tired so that I don't isolate myself from my children in order to rest. They know they can watch TV, play on the computer, and so forth, and I don't require them to be extra quiet. I do expect them not to wake me from a nap unless they need something. This has worked very well for several years.

A patient of mine with gait problems had a stair lift to get her up and down stairs. She complained that it was difficult to navigate once upstairs because her walker was downstairs. I suggested she buy or borrow a used walker for upstairs so one was always at hand. I had another patient make a dolly out of a used golf bag to carry out garbage, and so forth. Don't fight the disability—be creative in getting around it!

Insomnia is a frequent problem in the general population, and even more common in people with chronic illnesses. First, look for obvious causes. These include caffeine, stimulants, and pain. Sleep apnea, in which there are very brief periods of not breathing at night, can cause poor quality sleep and fatigue. Restless legs can impair sleep quality. An all night sleep study (polysomnogram) can yield valuable information about the causes of both insomnia and fatigue.

The primary treatment for insomnia is behavioral. Stimulus control treatment is simple and easy to use. You should go to bed at the same time every night and get up at the same time each morning regardless of how little sleep you get. If you wake up for more than 20 minutes, get out of bed and go into a different room. Come back to bed when you start to feel a little sleepy. Repeat as needed throughout the night. Get the TV, your computer, your bills, and so forth out of the bedroom. Bedrooms are only for sleep (and sex). Relaxation tapes may help you if you practice every day.

In general, sleeping medication should only be used for a short term so they you do not get tolerant to them (and they lose effectiveness). Newer sleeping agents, such as zolpidem (Ambien) are better tolerated than older sedatives. If you are using an older sedative, temezepam (Restoril) is preferred because it gets out of your body a little faster. Zaleplon (Sonata), which is already on the market, has the advantage of only lasting for about four hours, so it can be taken in the middle of the night if you wake up and can't get back to sleep; usually you will be quite alert come the morning. Ramelteon (Rozerem) is a new, novel sleeping agent that has no real risk of dependency, and eszopiclone (Lunesta) is also available and is considered safe for long-term use.

Flurazepam (Dalmane) lasts too long, and triazolam (Halcion) has had such adverse effects it is rarely used. Sometimes trazadone (Desyrel) is prescribed for sleep; it is an old antidepressant that makes you sleepy. Beside dizziness, men who take it should be aware of the rare side effect of priapism, which is a prolonged painful erection. This is a urological emergency, and you must go right to an emergency room. If medication treatment doesn't work, you may need surgery, which carries some risk of impotency.

Sometimes a bedtime dose of another medication, such as an anti-anxiety drug, antidepressant, or pain medication will be sufficient to help sleep.

IX
Dealing with Relationships and Sexuality

One day a physical therapist noticed my wedding ring as I was grasping the parallel bars. "Is that for real or a fake?" she asked, "I know some men who wear them to keep women from hitting on them." I just mumbled that mine was real, but what I really wanted to say was that being broke, unemployed, and a cripple would probably work just fine for chasing off women. I have had a real plunge in my self-esteem and body image since being ill, and as a psychiatrist I notice the subtle changes in relationships with my patients. In my wheelchair, men feel less threatened by me and some women feel more comfortable; people tend to see the crippled me as non-aggressive and non-sexual. I also notice that I have more difficulty talking with non-disabled friends and relatives and sometimes I close myself off and become more distant to people.

There are good studies on what happens to relationships when one member becomes disabled. A paper entitled: *Personal Relationships, Illness, and Disability* by Renee Lyons (Journal of Leasurability, Volume 26, Number 3, Summer 1999) reviews the literature and makes a number of important points:

- Chronic illness and disability is an interpersonal issue rather than an individual one and the quality of relationships is closely tied with adaptation to illness

- Good social supports (friends and family) really do make a big difference in how the ill person copes.

- The trajectory (or life path) of the entire family of a chronically ill patient is changed forever

- Not only can disabled people lose friends, they are afraid of being dumped by spouses and other loved ones

- Decreased contact with friends and relatives can ironically occur just when strong supports are most needed

- Our family tends to respond most to the crisis phase of an illness and much less to the more wearying longstanding chronic illness phase

- Communication with a chronically ill person is more difficult and many people avoid it or are uncomfortable trying it. At the same time there is a responsibility for the disabled person to learn to communicate their needs clearly

I sent Jeff, my third year medical student in to interview Valerie, a young woman with depression and abdominal pain that we thought might be from psychological causes. Five minutes later he came out of her room. He explained to me that it was impossible to interview her since she started retching and vomiting the minute he came in the room. "How did she make you feel?" I asked. Jeff said he thought that she was pretty sick. "But you didn't tell me how she made you feel," I said, "and I'm wondering if you didn't feel like you would chew your own arm off to get out of there!" Jeff laughed and acknowledged his dis-

comfort. "She feels terrible about herself," I said, "and if she unconsciously drives you away, it confirms her view of herself as disgusting and unlovable. Go back, and tell her you need to talk with her, and if she needs to vomit, you'll give her a basin, but you won't leave." Jeff came back half an hour later this time, reported that the talk went well, that she never vomited, and she asked him when his next visit would be. The urge to prove that we are unlovable based on no longer loving ourselves can be a major way to sabotage a relationship.

Clearly, we need our families and friends in order to cope. Historically, we are a culture that puts disabled people at the margin of society. Many years ago I worked at a chronic care hospital where all sorts of people were basically warehoused; my older patients today still fear "the nursing home" which meant being put away, with a loss of contact with family and a loss of personal space and freedom. If we want to avoid being isolated we need to make some extra effort.

- Tell people what sort of help you might need.

- If you are visiting someone or going to a party, inquire about handicapped accessibility issues in advance. The more you plan, the better things will go.

- Deal openly with the fact that you may not meet as many of your partner's needs as you did when you were well. Encourage your partner to get some of those needs met in another way.

- If you are suffering from fears of abandonment or being dumped, handle them in an adult way. Neither being overly needy or pushing the other person away by insisting you can do everything by yourself are particularly good ways of handling a relationship.

- Find activities you can still do with others in which being ill/disabled is not a major disadvantage.

- Learn coping skills so that your chronic pain doesn't end up causing chronic frustration in your relationships.

Sexual problems can be a major cause of distress in patients with peripheral neuropathy, even when normal sexual response is possible. Furthermore, there are pervasive social beliefs that disabled people are not interested in or not capable of sexual function. Finally, finding a willing partner may be harder for someone with a chronic medical illness.

There are a number of key myths about sex and disability: (parts of this list come from *"Speaking of Sex: Common Myths About Sex and Neuromuscular Disorders,"* by Margaret Wahl, Quest, Volume 4, Number 3,1997, An MDA Publication)

Myth #1—Disabled people are unattractive.

- **Fact**: Lots of fully able people are unattractive, and they have sex. Lots of disabled people are attractive. As one of my supervisors used to say: "love is blind, or no one would ever get married." We tend to view ourselves as unattractive, and then perpetuate this view to others, and then blame them for not finding us attractive.

Myth #2—People with neurological diseases lose sexual function.

- **Fact**: Many people with sensory or motor neuropathy have intact autonomic function necessary for sexual performance.

Myth #3—People with neuropathy lose interest in sex.

- **Fact**: While both illness and aging can decrease arousal and ability to have sex, loss of interest is not necessarily the case.

Myth #4—Sex is the only way to feel close to your partner.

- **Fact**: There are a lot of ways to feel intimate with others; you just never see them demonstrated on prime time TV.

Myth #5—Sexual abstinence can be harmful to you.

- **Fact**: Probably not harmful, but why take unnecessary chances?

Myth #6—No one will ever love me if I am disabled.

- **Fact**: No one will ever love you if you go around making up reasons for him or her not to love you. Otherwise, it's up to you. Remember, even Hitler had a girlfriend!

Myth #7—People with neuropathy are more comfortable sleeping alone.

- **Fact**: Many couples with a disabled partner end up in separate beds because of a breakdown in communication and mutual frustration. When I talk with a couple where one partner has a major illness, I always inquire about sleeping arrangements. Often taking separate beds or separate bedrooms is a negative way to cope with frustration and resentment in the relationship.

Myth #8—What worked before will still work now.

- **Fact**: You may have to make a lot of changes to have a good sex life. The neuropathy may cause fatigue and limit your ability to be acrobatic in bed. More foreplay and fantasy may be needed; Helen Kaplan Singer, the grandmother of sex therapy, once said, "sex is friction plus fantasy."

Myth #9—I won't be able to use my preferred sexual positions.

- **Fact**: The only critical sexual position is for you and your partner to be in the same room at the time of sex. Life changes things a lot—for a married couple with young children foreplay may consist of "quick honey, the kids are asleep."

If you are having problems with sex you should talk with a doctor who takes your concern seriously. Don't work with doctors who tell you that you have to give up sex or that your problem is "just part of your disease."

Sexual dysfunction in neuropathy can be from a number of causes. First, there are biological causes, such as nerve damage, blood vessel damage (for instance diabetes), and hormonal problems. Secondary biologic causes can include chronic pain and fatigue. A third biologic cause of dysfunction can be a side effect to medication. Psychological causes, including religious upbringing and body self-image can have a major impact on functioning. Finally social issues such as finding a partner and being comfortable with a disability can also impact sexual function.

It is easy to find the above causes in cases of neuropathy. Sometimes it is a result of damaged nerves, such as in diabetic neuropathy. Sexual problems can also be the result of fatigue, anxiety, depression, or just not feeling very appealing. Some medications you are taking may have sexual side effects. For example, the selective serotonin reuptake inhibitors (SSRIs), which include Prozac, Zoloft, Celexa, Lexapro, Paxil, and Luvox, can all cause problems with sexual interest, arousal, and orgasm function—they can prevent orgasms in women and prevent ejaculation in men. Many other medications, both psychiatric and for other diseases, have sexual side effects.

Psychiatrists often deal with the sexual side effects of depression or drugs used to treat depression. Medications such as bupropion, buspirone, and sildenafil (Viagra) may reverse sexual side effects. Viagra may be effective in men with a broad range of diseases including neuropathy. Two similar drugs, Levitra (vardenafil) and Cialis (tadalafil), are now on the market—Cialis has the advantage of lasting for more than a day after each dose. Older treatments for erectile dysfunction include injection into the penis of a prostaglandin. Vacuum pumps may help some men, and urologists can help decide who might benefit from penile implants. Certain hormones may end up being useful for men and women, although not standard therapy as yet. Arginine preparations, both taken by mouth and applied topically, have been reported to have some effect in sexual problems in women, although this is not proven. There is a prostaglandin in the medicine for men called "Muse" that may work for women. Sex is important to people, and more medicines will be developed. Even simple things, such as an adequate lubricant for women with vaginal dryness, may be very valuable. DO NOT GIVE UP—people have been able to have some kind of satisfying sex under every imaginable obstacle, including severe neurological problems such as spinal cord injury.

A good sexual history should include your past, your current sexual activity, your sexual preferences, and a good deal more. The history can provide a great deal of information that leads to proper diagnosis. For example, if a woman is only aroused by partners who are not her husband, this is a psychological and not a physical problem. Find a doctor who is comfortable talking about sex (psychiatrists, gynecologists, urologists, and marital and sex therapists may be good choices) and try to recover this part of your life. A good resource is *Enabling Romance: A Guide to Love, Sex, and Relationships for People* with Disabilities by Ken Kroll (http://www.newmobility.com—home) or purchase over the Internet at Amazon.com. Magazines that deal with disability, such as New Mobilities, and that deal with illness, such as Quest (for muscular dystrophy) frequently have articles about dating and sexuality. An excellent resource book is *The Ultimate Guide to Sex and Disability* (Miriam Kaufman MD, et. al., Cleis Press 2003)

There is an online (and actual) adult toy/book/video shop called www.comeasyouare.com run by one of the coauthors that is helpful to the needs of the disabled and lists many other useful resources. On the Internet, www.goaskalice.com and www.sexualhealth.com both have a wide variety of sex education topics. Finally, www.sexsupport.org has a huge collection of links dealing with sexuality and many different illnesses.

Improving sex despite illness:

1. Be open to the whole spectrum of sexual experience. Stop defining only penis in vagina intercourse as the only "real sex." The whole range of experience from masturbation to mutual masturbation to oral sex is open to you, and traditional intercourse may be tougher physically than these options, especially in the face of chronic illness.

2. Plan sex. Spontaneous sex is harder to accomplish since you may be tired or in pain a lot of the time. Try to rest before sex so you have some energy. If you take medication for pain, try to take a dose an hour or so before sex so that you get a peak effect during sex.

3. Use plenty of a water-based or silicone-based lubricant. This can help a lot, especially as a women in chronic pain (or fatigue) may have more difficulty with natural lubrication.

4. Consider vibrators and other sex toys, as well as adult videos, to enhance excitement, and to help do some of the "work" of sex for you.

5. Learn to talk openly with your partner about what you like and what turns you on. Good communication and open sharing of fantasy can make up for a lot of whatever you physically can't do anymore.

6. Once in a while, have sex first and enjoy it later. By this I mean that you may almost never feel "in the mood" if you have chronic pain or weakness. Allowing sex to happen anyway may give you some enjoyment once you get going, and there are so many barriers to sex sometimes you just have to go for it. At the worst, what have you got to lose by trying?

7. Try positions that minimize pain and fatigue. There are lots of books in the self-help section of the book store on sex and it can be useful to look at some of them, especially with your partner. Physical and occupational therapists often have resources for positioning disabled patients. Contact associa-

tions relevant to your illness and see if they have explicit information about positions and dealing with disability.

8. Be firm with your doctor and other health care providers that you want to talk with them about sexual health issues. Seek out providers who don't try to change the subject or get embarrassed easily.

X
Dealing with Existential Issues:
Why Me?

What I have learned from my experience with chronic illness thus far:

It's always darkest just before things turn utterly black.

Inside every dark cloud is a silver lining holding a potentially lethal lightning bolt.

Sometimes when God shuts a door, he also closes the window on your outstretched fingers.

In 1997 I came home from a cruise to find out a close friend of mine, a psychiatric nurse, had committed suicide. In the fall of that year I started the endless series of tests as my neuropathy progressed. During the same time my wife had a bleed in her eye and had heroic surgery to restore her eyesight. Over the last decade we faced my wife's treatment for thyroid cancer as well as repeated eye surgeries. My illness got to the point where I could no longer work nights and weekends and my employer used this as a reason to fire me—the ADA has very little protection if someone wants you gone. We went bankrupt and lost our house. My wife worked full time while fighting active rheumatoid arthritis while I learned to cope with at home duties. Of all the losses the one that most persistently plagues me is being too ill to practice. It took me twelve years of education (college, med school, residency) to be able to practice psychiatry and nine years into my career I was diagnosed with an incurable disease. Most people with my disease respond to a first line treatment; I failed all three. Without exaggeration I can tell you I have treated many people with life circumstances much tougher than mine. The courage and persistence I have witnessed in patients who have endured unspeakable trauma compels me to try to cope with my own situation. If my patients didn't give up hope, then I must try to carry on with some shred of dignity.

Sometimes I feel like someone reached their hand into my chest, pulled out my heart and is trying to feed it to me. I can't believe I am so sick that I can't practice psychiatry, which for me was an endless source of fascination and inspiration. I have read emails from many fellow sufferers. The level of personal faith and spirituality many of them have achieved astounds me. Not me. I survive through persistent pessimism, the idea that I better enjoy at least a little of today because things could, indeed, be worse tomorrow.

Life is full of luck, the vast majority of it bad. It is hard for me to think of examples of good luck besides something like winning the lottery. People often talk about their good luck but many times this is either "less bad luck than possible" or "good luck influenced by good work." Less bad luck than possible or "negative good luck" is often invoked. It may take the form of "you are very lucky you didn't die in the car crash even though you broke 8 ribs" or "you are lucky to still be alive." Most of this so-called good luck is simply not getting the worst possible outcome. But this is not truly good luck. Good luck would be having avoided the accident entirely.

Another kind of fake good luck, good luck influenced by work, is also often apparent. Many students have come to me and told me how lucky they are to have gotten a good grade on a final exam. If I ask them if they studied for the exam, they always tell me how hard they worked. Yet they still see their success as "good luck." I have also seen this in my chronically ill patients who battle terrific odds, manage to keep their lives together, and then remark to me that they have been "very lucky."

Often what we think of as bad luck is really bad people doing bad things to us. The fact that over a billion people don't have access to clean water isn't bad luck, it is bad government, and bad people not sharing resources. The lives of the ridiculously rich and overprivileged depend heavily on us common duffers accepting bad behavior as bad luck or ill fate. If we stop buying into this and actually want rich and powerful people to be accountable, a revolution would start.

So what do we make of a world in which bad luck is almost a certainty and good luck very much a long shot? Don't tell me how lucky I am, that it could be worse. Don't tell me that you admire my courage; I am not courageous, just trying to hang on for dear life. Don't tell me I'll grow from this experience, and don't tell me to stay hopeful. Don't tell me I don't look that bad. Don't tell me about someone you know who has it worse. Don't tell me that this is part of God's plan. Don't tell me that this could all be for the best, and don't tell me that things don't stink. My life would have been better if I had never gotten sick.

Almost everyone with a chronic illness struggles with the question of why this has happened to him or her. "Why me?" you ask yourself, "I'm not a bad person." We need to consider why bad things happen in the first place. My favorite explanation for this is that good and evil, and sickness and health are not related at all. That is, if God always rewarded good behavior and punished bad behavior, then being "good" would have no other meaning than sucking up to God to get a guaranteed reward. Being bad would just be stupid or masochistic, and there would be no way we could show that we are sincerely good for its own sake. Since we know that people can be good or bad under most circumstances, we know that being good is something we can do despite what has happened to us. Rabbi Harold Kushner, author of *Why Bad Things Happen to Good People*, said something to the effect that thinking that nothing bad will happen if you behave well is like thinking that a bull will not charge you because you are a vegetarian.

It is up to each of us with peripheral neuropathy to find our own answer to "why me?' Some people choose to believe that it is bad luck, others that it is God's will for them, others that it happened for some higher reason. You need to believe what makes sense to you and helps you cope.

A lot of times we don't really consider the meaning of life until life becomes bad. When I was still practicing psychiatry I knew the meaning of life. Life was getting up at 7 in the morning and seeing patients until 9 at night. If I worked hard, I could help some of them feel a little better. The meaning of life was to reduce some of the suffering in it and that was good enough for me. I even believed that psychiatric theory could give me a full understanding of the problems of the world and offer ways to deal with them. It wasn't until I had to stop practicing that I realized psychiatry couldn't be the entire answer. Now I have to search for a new meaning that is compelling enough to make it worth while getting up in the morning.

Cindy was a survivor of breast cancer, a young mother of two school-age boys. She had been through mastectomy, radiation, and chemo, and was being watched carefully for some suspicious bone lesions. Her oncologist referred her for treatment of depression. There is an old saying in psychiatry, "don't worry about saying the wrong thing, it can't possibly be worse than what the patient has already been through." Cindy and I played a game called "Dumbest Things People Said." Every week she would tell me the most useless or inconsiderate remarks people made to her regarding her cancer. This would lead to a discussion of what sort of advice and comfort did work for her. We were able to get past her guilt at no longer believing that "everything happens for a reason" and get to what beliefs and values she could still hold on to.

This is a technique I first learned from my Rabbi when I was 18 years old and came home from college to find my grandfather dying of lung cancer. Upset, I sought advice from my Rabbi, but I really expected little more than advice from the Bible and Talmud about how Jews deal with death. Instead he started out by saying: "when you first think about death, Scott, it seems as if God crapped all over the universe." Meeting someone emotionally where they are, rather than with theory or dogma is a remarkably effective way to make a connection. Note that he did not say that God did crap all over the universe, just that it must seem that way to me in all of my distress.

I should note that acknowledging that a situation sucks should be a first step in trying to cope with the problem at hand. This acknowledgement in no way entitles the patient to give up, become a professional victim, or deny responsibility for themselves. Hopefully making a realistic assessment of the severity of the situation will help the patient, as well as family and friends, mobilize in useful ways.

There are times I tell my patients that since there may not be a satisfactory answer to "why me?" that it will be more helpful to move on to another question.

That question is, what do I do now that I have the illness? Viktor Frankl, a psychiatrist and concentration camp survivor, gives some good answers to this question in his book *Man's Search for Meaning*. Frankl says that we can find meaning in life through work, love, and suffering. Frankl in no way suggests that suffering is good—in fact he stresses that if pain can be relieved it should be, and not doing so is crazy. However, if the suffering can't be removed, than meaning can be found in what one does or accomplishes despite the suffering. Even in severely disabled patients, meaning and worth can be found in one's attitude toward the suffering—do you focus on the suffering or on other aspects of your life besides the suffering? Frankl in no way suggests this is easy, but I believe he is sincere and perhaps correct when I read the first part of his book detailing his three years in Nazi death camps. During an attack of typhus, he was ill and near death, and scribbled notes for his book anyway, so that if he survived he would have a story to tell, and in fact he did survive. Frankl quotes Nietsche who said: He who has a **why** to live can bear almost any **how**.

Frankl looks at three aspects of suffering: pain, guilt, and the inevitability of death. Pain can only be lessened but not usually removed in neuropathy, but every aspect should be made to improve the pain. The patient must also find meaningful things to focus attention on that are not pain. I have found that this also helps relieve the pain. I have noticed that I experience very little fatigue or leg pain while in with a patient, but when there is a break or the day is over I am much more consciously aware of the discomfort. This is supported by theories of pain and what may block it. For example, there is a study that shows that soldiers inflicted with gunshot wounds need fewer painkillers than civilians with similar wounds. The soldiers, perhaps, are trained to expect and handle pain.

Guilt, the second aspect of suffering, can be dealt with by improving our behavior. Guilt figures in neuropathy when we feel bad that we are putting our families through this, or when we behave more poorly because we are tired and frustrated. Guilt can go away when we stop the behavior that makes us feel guilty. For example, if you tend to take out your pain on others by being crabby, and you chose to go to therapy to work on this, not only will your relationships probably improve but you will also stop feeling so guilty.

Death, the third aspect of suffering, also needs to be confronted. Death can be a way of reminding us to make the most of our lives. Frankl suggests that you "live as if you were living for the second time and had acted as wrongly the first time as you are about to act now."

This gives us a chance to evaluate and change our behavior on a daily basis. Think about this for a second. Not only does it apply to situations regarding others, such as trying not to be grumpy around friends, it also applies to us neuropathy sufferers. If you had treated yourself poorly in your "first life" by being overstressed, overworked, or not taking time for yourself, then this is a chance to correct it. In my second life I go for physical therapy three times a week and I do a progressive relaxation exercise every day. When I was working full time as a psychiatrist, I would work to the point of exhaustion and then come home and fall asleep. So in my new life I have had the chance to correct bad habits that I would not have if I disobeyed Frankl's dictum.

Uncertain outcomes, pain, disability, chronicity, and *incurability* are all characteristics of neuropathy. Each contributes to the burden of suffering: Yet through our own actions we may be able to decrease our suffering. While we can't control everything that happens to us, we can control our own behavior and deal with these issues.

- *Uncertainty*—Everyone lives with uncertainty, they just don't know it. Chronically ill patients can't forget it. We need to learn to live in the present, which can be so hard that it deserves its own book. To paraphrase a famous Rabbi: "change yourself one day before you die." Since you don't know when that day will come, you need to make changes every day to follow this advice.

- *Pain*—Physical and emotional pain should be treated; see a psychologist, psychiatrist, pain specialist, or rehabilitation doctor (physiatrist). Don't ever give up looking for treatments for the pain! The search itself is part of the treatment—people who give up probably experience more pain, as well as anxiety and depression, than those who don't.

- *Disability*—Loss of previous roles and physical abilities—search for something you can do (I discussed this earlier).

- *Chronicity*—Waking up each morning knowing the illness will still be there requires making the effort to have something pleasurable planned each day.

- *Incurability*—Holding on to wishes that you would just magically get better. Give up fantasies of being rescued or getting better and deal with the fact that this is how things will be. This will give you more freedom to pursue a richer life.

Coping with peripheral neuropathy is no easy task. As you have read in these pages, and as you have no doubt experienced, these illnesses can affect every part of your life. Learning how to deal is hard. You will need to see which suggestions printed here and elsewhere are actually helpful to you. You will have to create your own style of coping. This is a hard journey on a trip you never asked to go on. Still I believe there is reason for hope. The speed of medical progress is faster than ever before and there is good reason to believe that newer treatments will be available in our lifetimes. The current treatments for pain, fatigue, depression, and anxiety are often quite good. No matter what the illness, people feel better when these issues are addressed.

There is even more reason to be hopeful leaving aside what modern medicine can offer you. Over years of practicing psychiatry I have always been amazed at the ability of people to recover from tragedy and trauma. Sometimes they do this with my help, sometimes they do it on their own and I simply bear witness to it. I used to joke with my medical students that "despite the best medical care the patient got better and was sent home from hospital recovered." It is a spiritual experience for me to watch people endure and get past agonies that I can barely imagine. I have seen a patient suicidal from severe chronic pain with no known cause who three years later I met at the gym where she was working out, pain free, happy and smiling. Everyone with severe neuropathy knows despair at some point. We ask ourselves why we have to suffer so and whether we are worthwhile, whether life is worth living like this, and whether or not we should just give up. The trick is to not give up even when things seem hopeless. Just because you feel hopeless now doesn't mean you will always feel that way. I am not trying to suggest in the least that coping is easy, just that it is possible. I don't always know why my patients start to cope better, just that most of them do. I think we have an innate tendency toward health and coping. When you feel that you can't cope, you can "borrow" some hope from others. I have told many patients with severe depression that I don't expect them to feel hopeful; in fact that I know that they can't feel hopeful because hopelessness is part of their illness. I just ask them to believe that **I feel hopeful about them**, based on my experience in dealing with people who feel hopeless.

Maimonides, a famous Rabbi and physician, wrote a prayer for doctors in which he asks that "in the sufferer, may I always see the human being." I think that it is hard to see our own humanness under the pile of EMG test results and medications, but your own humanness is always there. No one and no disease can take it away from you. You may lose sight of it, and so may your doctors, but it is there. Peripheral neuropathy, like all illnesses, poses a threat to your humanness, ultimately the only threat of any final importance. When you rediscover your personal identity, your self worth, your uniqueness, your ability to relate to others, then you have beaten the illness whether or not you are in remission. Your journey will be hard, the road will be painful, the tasks demanding, and the time short, but this is the essence of all existence. You have plenty of company and you will meet other travelers along the way. Life is about the journey, not the outcome. I wish you Godspeed.

Resource Directory

The Neuropathy Association; www.neuropthy.org (for patients), or www.neuropathy.com (the neuropathy store), and www.neuropathymd.org (for doctors)

You can contact them by email at info@neuropathy.org, by telephone
at 1-800-247-6968 or 212-692-0662, or by mail by writing to:
The
Neuropathy Association
The Lincoln Building
60 E. 42nd Street
Suite 942
New York City, NY 10165-0999

The Jack Miller Center at University of Chicago: www.millercenter.uchicago.edu

Neuromuscular Web Site of the University of Washington, St. Louis: at: www.neuro.wustl.edu/neuromuscular

Sexuality and disability: www.sexualhealth.com Lots of resources and articles specific to medical problems

Go Ask Alice at www.goaskalice.com Thousands of questions and answers about sex

Good Vibrations 1-800-289-8423, www.goodvibes.com (well known sex product catalog)

Enabling Romance: A Guide to Love, Sex, and Relationships for People with Disabilities (and the People who Care About Them) by Ken Kroll and Erica Levy Klein, 1992, No Limits Communications—also has website: http://www. newmobility.com—home

Peripheral Neuropathy Medical Information at Medline Plus: http://medlineplus.nlm.nih. gov/medlineplus/peripheralnervedisorders.html Neuromuscular disease information

JoAnn LeMaistre: Synopsis of her work on coping with chronic illness   at: http://www.alpineguild.com/COP-ING%20WITH%20CHRONIC%20ILLNESS.htm

Numb Toes and Aching Soles: Coping with Peripheral Neuropathy by John A. Senneff (paperback—July 1999)

Numb Toes and Other Woes: More on Peripheral Neuropathy
by John A. Senneff (Paperback—July 2001)

Nutrients for Neuropathy (The Numb Toes Series, Vol 3)
by John A. Senneff, Laurence J. Kinsella (Paperback—July 2002)

After the Diagnosis: From Crisis to Personal Renewal for Patients With Chronic Illness

by JoAnn LeMaistre Ph. D. (Paperback—November 1995)

The Chronic Illness Workbook: Strategies and Solutions for Taking Back Your Life—by Patricia A. Fennell; Paperback

Full Catastrophe Living: Using the Wisdom of Your Body and Mind to Face Stress, Pain, and Illness

by Jon Kabat-Zinn, et al (Paperback) (Dr. Kabat-Zinn's Mindfulness Meditation Workshops at University of Massachusetts Medical Center are internationally acclaimed for their effectiveness in treating chronically ill patients)

Living With Chronic Illness: Days of Patience and Passion

by Cheri Register

Essential Guide to Chronic Illness: The Active Patient's Handbook

by James W. Long

One More Day: Daily Meditations for People With Chronic Illness (Hazelden Medition Series)

by Safra Kobrin Pitzele, Sefra Kobrin Pitzele

Beyond Chaos: One Man's Journey Alongside His Chronically Ill Wife

by Gregg Piburn (Paperback—May 1999)

Sick and Tired of Feeling Sick and Tired: Living with Invisible Chronic Illness, Second Edition

by Paul J. Donoghue, Mary Elizabeth Siegel (Paperback—July 2000)

Living Well: A Twelve-Step Response to Chronic Illness and Disability

by Martha Cleveland

Above and Beyond: 365 Meditations for Transcending Chronic Pain and Illness

by J. S. Dorian, P. S. Dorian (Paperback—June 1996)

Chronically Happy: Joyful Living In Spite Of Chronic Illness

by Lori Hartwell (Paperback)

Surviving Your Spouse's Chronic Illness

by Chris McGonigle

<u>Kitchen Table Wisdom: Stories That Heal</u>
by Rachel Naomi Remen (Paperback—August 1997)

<u>In Pain?: A Self-help Guide for Chronic Pain Sufferers</u>
by Chris Wells, Graham Nown

<u>Chronic Illness and the Twelve Steps: A Practical Approach to Spiritual Resilience</u>
by Martha Cleveland (**Paperback**)

<u>Finding the Joy in Today: Practical Readings for Living With Chronic Illness</u>
by Sefra Kobrin Pitzele (Paperback)

<u>SELF-CARE NOW! 30 TIPS TO HELP YOU TAKE CARE OF YOURSELF WHEN CHRONIC ILLNESS TURNS YOUR LIFE UPSIDE DOWN</u>
BY PAULINE SALVUCCI (PAPERBACK)

<u>Living Better: Every Patient's Guide to Living with Illness</u>
by Carol J. Langenfeld, et al (**Paperback**)

On the next pages are worksheets you can carry with you at all times and bring to each doctor's appointment. Copy them and try using them!

Worksheet for Neuropathy Patients

NAME: _____ **Date of Birth:** _____

Social Security #: _____

Address: _____

Insurance Carrier: _____

Group # _____

Patient ID #: _____

Plan # _____

Insurance Phone # (to precertify coverage): _____

Emergency Contact: _____

Phone: _____

☐ My working diagnosis is:

_____

☐ My neurologist is:

_____

☐ My hospital is:

_____

UPCOMING APPOINTMENTS:

DATE	TEST	RESULT
Blood tests		
EMG		
Spinal tap		
MRIs		
Evoked Potentials		
Other		

Treatments:

DATE	TREAT-MENT	DOSE	RESULT	SIDE EFFECTS	NEXT TREAT-MENT DATE

NOTES & COMMENTS:

OTHER MEDICAL PROBLEMS

Problem	Started	Doctor treating it	Doctor's phone #

ALLERGIES & SENSITIVITIES: →→→		Pharmacy:	Phone:

PRESCRIPTION MEDICATIONS	DOSE	HOW OFTEN I TAKE IT	REASON I TAKE IT

OVER THE COUNTER MEDICATION	HERBAL MEDICATION	VITAMINS	NUTRITIONAL SUPPLEMENTS

Survival Rules for Peripheral Neuropathy

☐ I will go to my neurologist on a regular basis

☐ I will insist on a second opinion if there is doubt about my diagnosis

☐ I will make sure I understand the risks, benefits, and alternatives for any proposed treatments

☐ I will call my doctor or go to the emergency room for any sudden change in symptoms

☐ I will insist on immediate treatment for any new problems

☐ I will take my medicine as directed

☐ I will tell my doctors about any alternative, complementary, or herbal remedies I am using

☐ I will make sure I understand what my doctor explains to me or ask for more explanation

☐ I will seek psychological counseling or psychiatric care if I find it difficult to cope

☐ I will seek counseling if my illness starts to interfere with my relationships

☐ I will ask for repeat testing if my condition changes

☐ I will appeal any denials by my insurance company for diagnostic tests or treatment for neuropathy

PLEASE CONTRIBUTE TO THE NEXT EDITION OF:
COPING WITH PERIPHERAL NEUROPATHY

Send your personal stories, ideas, coping tips, information, resource information, websites, suggestions for additional material and topics, requests for future topics to:

E-mail: sibshrink225@msn.com

OR

Scott Berman MD
Good Shepherd Plaza
Att: Rehability—SB
850 S. Fifth St.
Allentown, PA 18103

All submissions used in subsequent editions will credit you by name (unless you ask to remain anonymous).

Thank you in advance for your help in creating a more thorough guide for future patients!

About the Author

Scott I Berman MD, FAPA, received his undergraduate degree in Biomedical Ethics from Brown University. He attended medical school at Virginia Commonwealth University, and served a four-year psychiatric residency at Hahnemann University Hospital in Philadelphia, PA.

Dr. Berman went on to direct an inpatient psychiatric unit, develop a gero-med-psych program, and direct a Day Hospital. His interests include psychiatric treatment of the medically ill (psychosomatic medicine), psychodynamic psychotherapy, and psychopharmacology. In 1998, at the age of 40, he was diagnosed with the neuropathy CIDP (chronic inflammatory demyelinating polyneuropathy). He lives in Bethlehem PA with his wife Jennifer, his three children, Rachel, Josh, and Jordan, and their dog, Willie. Doctor Berman has done extensive teaching and lecturing in psychiatry as well as in psychosocial issues in treating peripheral neuropathy.

978-0-595-44967-5
0-595-44967-0